Health, Place and Society

Health, Place and Society

Mary Shaw

Department of Social Medicine, University of Bristol

Danny Dorling

School of Geography, University of Leeds

Richard Mitchell

Research Unit in Health, Behaviour and Change, University of Edinburgh

Preface by Peter Haggett

An imprint of Pearson Education

Harlow, England • London • New York • Reading, Massachusetts • San Francisco • Toronto • Don Mills, Ontario • Sydney •
Tokyo • Singapore • Hong Kong • Seoul • Taipei • Cape Town • Madrid • Mexico City • Amsterdam • Munich • Paris • Milan

For Robbie Dorling, born 3 June 2001.

Pearson Education Limited
Edinburgh Gate
Harlow
Essex CM20 2JE

and Associated Companies throughout the world

Visit us on the World Wide Web at:
www.pearsoneduc.com

First edition published in Great Britain in 2002

ISBN 0 130 16455 0

British Library Cataloguing-in-Publication Data
A catalogue record for this book is available from the British Library

Library of Congress Cataloging-in-Publication Data
A catalog record for this book is available from the Library of Congress

10 9 8 7 6 5 4 3 2 1
07 06 05 04 03 02

Typeset in 11/12 pt Adobe Garamond by 63
Produced by Pearson Education Asia Pte Ltd.
Printed in Singapore

Contents

Contents

Preface

The history of most university institutions shows a few rare but productive periods when a small group of scholars come briefly together to strike sparks from each other to ignite a new flame of research. I'm proud that the Bristol Department of Geography has, over its eighty years, shown a number of such episodes when clusters in both physical and human geography have critically taken off. The late 1990s were such an episode when Danny Dorling, Mary Shaw, and Richard Mitchell came briefly together to study social and spatial health inequalities.

I had met Danny a decade before as external examiner of his remarkable doctoral thesis in geography and mathematics at the University of Newcastle, where he showed an astonishing Edward Tufte-like flair for conveying critical ideas in social geography by the most innovative of visual displays in quantitative information. He joined the Bristol staff in 1996 after holding a British Academy Research Fellowship and is now a professor at Leeds. Mary joined him at Bristol the following year, bringing deep skills in sociology and social research, and with experience of research and teaching in both the Czech Republic and Australia. Richard joined the team in 1999 from London, bringing valuable skills in GIS and housing needs.

This talented team has now joined forces in this innovative text for students in the social and health sciences who are interested in contemporary medical geography and medical sociology. It provides a valuable historical perspective on health, place and society, and introduces the new ways of mapping and measuring them. It illustrates the social and spatial patterning of health and shows how health inequalities arise and the role of spatial mobility in shaping the pattern. Finally, it provides an historical perspective on medical mapping from the mid-nineteenth century to the start of the new century. All the chapters are marked by innovative teaching methods and a wide range of well-researched examples at a variety of geographical scales. That this is no dull textbook is shown by the sheer variety of sources used, with novels and films as well as scientific works as recommended 'reading'.

More than most texts this is, I believe, a very personal work. One cannot read it without sensing the authors' zest for their chosen field, and a refusal to be hidebound by disciplinary boundaries or conventions. It simply bubbles with their shared interest and enthusiasm for their subject and their wish to see it at work on the health problems that loom all around us. In short, it is the kind of book which, from the quiet waters of retirement, makes me wish I was starting out as an undergraduate again. It deserves to be widely used.

Peter Haggett
Institute for Advanced Studies
University of Bristol

Acknowledgements

The authors would like to thank the following people for their invaluable assistance in the preparation of this book: Alison Dorling, Carol Emslie, Drew Ellis, Ben Joyner, Helen Lambert, Jonathan Tooby, Helena Tunstall and Lois Wright.

We are particularly grateful to Peter Haggart for his kind preface and to Matthew Smith and Liz Tarrant at Pearson Education.

We are grateful to the following for permission to reproduce copyright material:

Figure 2.4 from http://www.spartacus.schoolnet.co.uk/IRinspectors.htm; Figure 3.4 Mortality Statistics Series DHI No. 29, National Statistics © Crown Copyright 2000; Figure 3.6 from http://www-dceg.ims.mci.nih.gov/atlas/index.html; Box 3.17 extract from freelands/co.uk/e-coli.htm; Figure 3.7 from http://www-viz.tamu.edu/faculty/house/cartograms/1996Cartogram.html; Table 4.5 is reprinted with permission from Elsevier Science (*The Lancet*, 1997, Vol. 350, pp. 383–8, Leon *et al.*); Figure 5.2 from data from E.O. Lawrence Berkeley National Laboratory High-radon Project; Figure 6.3 British Medical Journal (1999) *BMJ*, 318, 10th April and Figure 7.8 Forster, F. (1996) Use of a demographic base map for the presentation of areal data in epidemiology, *British Journal of Preventative and Social Medicine*, 20: 165–171, both BMJ Publishing Group; Figure 7.5 Taylor, I. (1955) An epidemiology map. *Ministry of Health Monthly Bulletin*, 14, 200–1, and Figure 7.13 Mitchell, R., Dorling, D. and Shaw, M. (2000) *Inequalities in Life and Death: What if Britain were More Equal?*, Bristol/York: The Policy Press/Joseph Rowntree Foundation, reproduced by kind permission. Material in Box 2.5 adapted from Fisher, P. and Ward, A. (1994) Medicine in Europe; complementary medicine in Europe, *BMJ*, 309: 107–11, BMJ Publishing Group. Box 2.5 adapted from Medicine in Europe in *BMJ* 309, BMJ Publishing Group (Fisher, P. and Ward, A. 1994); Box 3.3 from *Living in Britain – Results from the 1998 General Household Survey* (ONS 2000), Figure 4.6 from *Mortality Statistics Series DH1 No.29* (ONS 1997), Table 4.6 from *Health Statistics Quarterly 7* (Fitzpatrick and Kelleher 2000), Box 4.8 from Appendix A: sources and methods in *Health Inequalities: Decennial Supplement* edited by F. Drever and M. Whitehead, The Stationery Office (Bunting, J. 1997) and Figure 7.5 from *Ministry of Health Monthly Bulletin 14* (1955), all Crown copyright, Crown copyright material is reproduced under Class Licence number CO1W0000039 with the permission of the Controller of HMSO and the Queen's Printer for Scotland; Figure 3.5 from http://www.devon.gov.uk/dris/commstat/depr_mnu.html, copyright Devon County Council; Figure

4.3 from Ben Joyner; Table 4.3 from United Nations Development Programme *Human Development Report, 1999*, published by Oxford University Press, New York, reprinted by permission of UNDP (UNDP 2000); Figure 4.4 after Leading causes of death (%) in the rich and poor areas of the world, 1997 in *Burdens of Disease 1997*, World Health Organization (WHO 1998); Figure 4.5 after Outbreaks of infectious disease with more than 10,000 cases, 1970-1990's in *Removing Obstacles to Healthy Development*, World Health Organization (WHO 1998); Table 4.8 from Occupational class and cause specific mortality in middle aged men in 11 European countries: comparison of population based studies in *BMJ* 316, BMJ Publishing Group (Kunst, A. *et al.* 1998); Box 5.17 from Income inequality and mortality: importance to health of individual income, psychosocial environment, or material conditions in *BMJ* 320, BMJ Publishing Group (Lynch, J. *et al.* 2000); Box 5.9 from Radiation Reassessed; Figure 6.3 from Editor's Choice in *BMJ* 318, 10 April 1999, BMJ Publishing Group; Figure 7.1 after *Early Thematic Mapping in the History of Cartography*, University of Chicago Press (Robinson, A. H. 1982); Figure 7.8 from Use of a demographic base map for the presentation of areal data in epidemiology in *British Journal of Preventative and Social Medicine* 20, BMJ Publishing Group (Forster, F. 1966); Figure 7.9 from *National Atlas of Disease Mortality in the United Kingdom*, copyright 1970 by the Royal Geographical Society (Howe, G. M. 1970); Figure 7.12 reprinted from Transformations of maps to investigate clusters of diseases in *Social Science and Medicine*, Vol. 26, with permission from Elsevier Science, copyright 1988 (Selvin *et al.* 1988); and Figure 7.13 after *Inequalities in Life and Death: What if Britain Were More Equal?*, copyright The Policy Press and Joseph Rowntree Foundation, reprinted by permission of The Policy Press (Mitchell, R. *et al.* 2000).

While every effort has been made to trace the owners of copyright material, in a few cases this has proved impossible and we take this opportunity to offer our apologies to any copyright holders whose rights we may have unwittingly infringed.

Chapter 1

Introduction

What is this book about?

Have you ever thought about why some people are healthier and live longer than others? Unless you have never had the opportunity to go somewhere other than your immediate area of residence, you are bound to have noticed how different places vary, in terms of factors such as the housing you see (its design, size and quality), the facilities there (parks, shops, cinemas, factories) and the people (tall, short, fat, scruffy, happy or sad). You may also be aware that people vary as well: some smoke, some don't; some are rich and some poor; some live alone and others share their home with members of their family, or with friends. This book is about bringing these issues together – how people, places and health vary, and how they interact. The book is thus about social and spatial aspects of health – how and why health can vary between different places and different social groups.

In reading this book (as well as doing the related reading and activities we suggest) you will learn not only about a range of topics and themes, but also about the disciplines that we refer to here as 'medical geography' and 'medical sociology'. You will begin to find out about different perspectives (ways of looking at the world) different ways of gathering information (research sources and methods) and some of the ways that we can interrogate data in order to answer our research questions (types of analysis). We have endeavoured to write the book in a style that will appeal to anyone interested in learning about the world around them – so while it is substantively about issues surrounding health, many of the principles and practices could be applied to other topic areas. It is as much about provoking thought as about passing on knowledge.

There is also a strong element of time in the book – how patterns have changed over time (or remained the same) and how people move through space over time. We look at how health has been viewed and researched in different ways at different times and in different places by different people. We are interested in how health might be improved and how variations in health might be reduced in the future, on a worldwide scale, in particular countries and in particular localities. To think about how to achieve those aims a good starting point is to see how people have studied health in the past and compare that with how social scientists research health today. We ask whether we are gaining a better understanding of the determinants of health and introduce you to many current debates at the crossroads of medical geography and medical sociology.

Who is this book for?

This book is primarily written for undergraduate students of geography and sociology, but will also be relevant for those studying social sciences more generally, and for those studying and interested in health-related areas (medicine, nursing, public health and the caring professions). It is also a book for people who are interested in how researchers think. The three authors of this book are all actively involved in producing research papers and reports on health. However, when we write these papers and reports we rarely get a chance to describe how we view the larger picture – how we think all this work fits together. If you think that you might like to study issues around health and the social sciences further in the future, this book should give you an idea of the kinds of debates that are currently raging and of how a group of three people involved in those debates see the study of medical geography and sociology progressing.

What does the book aim to do?

The book has been written as an introduction to some of the themes, methods and thinking of contemporary medical geography and medical sociology. We have tried to do this in a novel and imaginative way. To do this we sometimes jump between themes and ideas, which you may find disconcerting, but perseverance will pay off as you begin to glimpse the wider picture we are trying to paint. The book aims to give you an idea of how disparate areas of the study of health in the social sciences fit together. We have incorporated pictures, cartoons, stories, films, novels and anything else we could think of to try to achieve our aims. This makes our book slightly unconventional.

While we aim to cover some central contemporary themes – such as health inequalities – we have tried not to do so in the same way that they have been covered in other textbooks. For example, most textbooks that discuss health inequalities almost always structure their coverage in the same way (covering artefact, health selection, behavioural and material explanations), but we take a different approach. You will end up learning similar things, but you will have got there by a different, hopefully more stimulating, path.

We have particularly tried to convey ideas both about how single research projects are conducted and how bodies of research develop and issues are debated among researchers. By the end of the book you should have a real feel for how research is done; you may even want to move on to conducting your own research projects. We also hope to give you an idea of how much work remains to be done and of how much we do not yet know about how society, geography and health are interconnected.

This book does not aim or claim to be a comprehensive, encyclopaedic guide either by topic, author or perspective. We pick and choose examples that highlight the processes of understanding that we are hoping to foster. For example, we have spent a lot of time covering issues of wealth, poverty and social class, writing less on issues of gender and very little on ethnicity. Where we spend less time on what we consider to be important topics, we guide you to further reading sources.

Similarly, we have not tried to write a handbook of methods for researching social and spatial aspects of health. We have chosen to cover only quantitative methods, not because we think they are more valuable than qualitative techniques, but because this is our main area of expertise. Nor have we tried to cover all aspects and forms of quantitative methods (there are many methods books for that), but rather we introduce some key basics that will help you get off to a solid start and highlight the techniques researchers actually use rather than those generally taught to undergraduate students.

While there are some similarities in the way the chapters are organized we have not aimed to provide a formulaic structure for each. We hope that this makes the book a less monotonous read. Each chapter was written by one of us, revised by another and further revised by the other (sometimes many times over) until we could all agree on what we wanted to say. We had some arguments and disagreements in writing this book but we eventually (mostly) agreed with what was finally said. The final product is the synthesis of three people's views, rather than an uncritical collection of them, and in the same vein we would encourage you to cast a critical eye as you read this and other sources.

What's in the book?

There are six substantive chapters which are divided into two sections. The first section (Chapters 2, 3 and 4) focuses on learning evidence, concepts, methods and analysis – acquiring tools of the trade. In the second section (Chapters 5, 6 and 7) the emphasis is more on looking at particular topics and working through research examples – using those tools. Below we provide a brief summary of each chapter so that even if you are just glancing at this book you can read the next couple of pages and get an idea of what the book is about. Hopefully after that you might like to read further.

Chapter 2 Health, place and society: an historical perspective

In this chapter we begin by asking: why take an historical perspective? We first discuss health in pre-modern societies and traditional medicine, and the plague in medieval Europe (its spread, responses to it and its consequences). We then move on to consider industrialization, urbanization and the rise of scientific medicine, looking at how these developments influenced science and medicine in general, and public health in particular. We then turn to the development of geographical and sociological thinking regarding health, concentrating on the study of suicide by Emile Durkheim and using this as an introduction to seeing variations in health as a combination of individual acts and social facts. We close with an overview of the centuries of change that have been covered and discuss where there has been continuity and where we can see a real break with the past.

Chapter 3 Mapping and measuring

We introduce this chapter by considering the characteristics of people that affect health and asking whether we should study risk at the individual or group level. We discuss the key variables of age, sex and wealth, as well as considering life course perspectives and clinical measures. We move on to consider the impact of where people live, in terms of 'space and place' and 'time and space'. We then consider data sources: censuses, surveys and routinely recorded data, before asking how these data can by analysed: considering the recoding of variables, deriving indicators and conducting statistical tests. We end the chapter looking at how these data can be mapped, including chloropleth maps, cartograms and point mapping techniques.

Chapter 4 The social and spatial patterning of health

In this chapter we begin with the global picture, covering causes of death across the world, looking at mortality by age and by sex and considering averages, variation and exceptions to the rule. We look at countries in one region of the world, examining recent mortality trends in eastern and central Europe, and considering the possible role of pollution, the collapse of health services, 'unhealthy' behaviours – smoking, alcohol and diet – and social and socio-economic factors. Next we turn to health at the regional and the local scales and their interaction with socio-economic factors. We discuss the size of class differences in mortality in different parts of Europe, the 'north/south divide' in Britain and specifically consider the influence of unemployment, social class and social capital on influencing patterns of health and illness. We conclude at the smallest geographical scale with some case studies of health in particular communities.

Chapter 5 Health inequalities: composition or context?

In this chapter we introduce the debate over composition and context and ask why health inequalities are important as a matter of equality and in terms of particular policy implications. We provide four examples of research projects that have tried to find evidence for the importance of context and show how their results differ because of the differing techniques which are used and the varying standpoints which are initially taken. We discuss the mechanisms that might be operating: the physical and environmental context, and the social context (including the tangible, state and social fabric of places). We end by asking to what extent it might be possible in the future to untangle the influences of context and composition in producing health outcomes and present the conundrum that this debate is itself influenced by our next major topic – mobility. Just when you think you are getting to grips with one of the social/geographical determinants of health you often find that it in turn is influenced by another determinant.

Chapter 6 Health and social/spatial mobility

Here we introduce issues relating to the impact of migration, immigration and social mobility on health. We show how a typology of movements can be constructed into which different kinds of mobility can be placed in order to try to ascertain their particular impact on patterns of health. We then cover each type of movement in turn, beginning with social class and social mobility (social immigration, class formation and small-scale internal social movements), moving on to geographical mobility (immigration, colonization and migration at both the macro- and micro-scales). We end this discussion by looking at how these two forms of movement combine to create a socio-spatial mobility that impacts upon health in the round. We conclude by turning the question on its head and considering how health can in turn affect mobility. We argue that a full understanding of how health variations are affected by context and composition is only possible if mobility is considered. How people and places change over time is a factor that both helps to create and maintain differences in their health.

Chapter 7 Putting research into context: from cholera to good health for all

In our final chapter we take an historical tour through the mapping of disease, moving from the mapping of cholera in the middle of the nineteenth century to the use of cartograms at the end of the twentieth century. We revisit many of the topics, concepts, methods and perspectives of the preceding chapters. We reiterate the importance of an historical perspective and a sense of 'what has gone before'. We see again elements of the social and spatial patterning of health and illness. We think once more about how diseases can be measured and mapped and about the patterns of health inequalities that we see as a consequence. Issues of composition and context, migration and mobility are never far from the frame. This last chapter is thus about how different researchers have mapped disease and mortality in different times and in different places, but it is also about how we need to appreciate that research has been conducted within different contexts. All interpretations of the world, including our own, need to be seen as 'of their time and place'. We finish the chapter by outlining the key messages that we hope this book has conveyed.

In all the chapters outlined above we include many examples, often drawing on studies from around the world. However, you will notice that our own national background is understandably over-represented. We are not trying to excuse this, but see it as a reflection of how the research world operates. Similarly, we have tried to explain how research, and thus knowledge, is affected by ideology, and at times we have been open about our own perspectives and

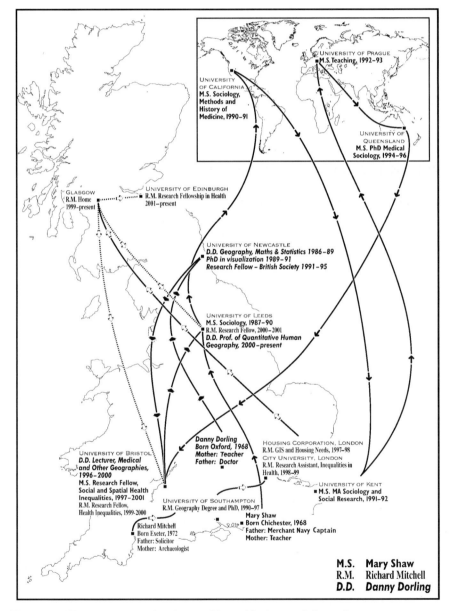

Figure 1.1 Where we are coming from: a biographical map of the authors.

position. At other times we might well have tried to present our particular views as 'general knowledge'! This is one of the reasons people write textbooks – they want to influence how other people view the world. Figure 1.1 will give you some indication of 'where we are coming from', both geographically and socially.

To counteract our indiscretions and particular idiosyncrasies, at the end of each chapter we suggest further reading, and also activities, which are designed as an extension of the knowledge and reasoning of the chapter. The only way in which you will be able to form a view of what the biases of this particular book are is by reading other similar books. We hope we have been more open than most in pointing out that any textbook comes with a particular set of preconceived assumptions that are not necessarily made clear in its text. Read this with an open mind and do not necessarily believe everything we say – we could be wrong – but also do not necessarily dismiss ideas you do not immediately accept – think 'why would they be arguing that?'

What we hope this book will achieve

We have already said what we hope you will get out of this book, in terms of understanding this topic. However, we also hope to encourage you to become more aware of the world around you – to encourage you to ask questions and look critically, we show you how to make your argument, and how to accept that you might not always be right!

Health matters. Having, and continuing to enjoy, good health is one of the aspects of life that is held most dearly by people all over the world – although most people in more affluent places realize this only when they fall ill. The study of health is a microcosm of the study of human lives in general – picking on one particularly emotive and important aspect of our lives. Through studying health we can increase our understanding of society more generally. The same methods that are used to ask why different people suffer different rates of illness can be applied to areas as wide ranging as the study of education, employment, housing, income and wealth – just to take a few examples. Issues of equality, definition, measurement, composition, context and mobility affect all of these and other aspects of our lives. Begin with health, but keep thinking more widely – why are things the way they are? Does it have to be this way?

SECTION I

Chapter 2

Health, place and society: an historical perspective

Chapter summary

In this chapter we begin by asking: why take an historical perspective? We first discuss health in pre-modern societies and traditional medicine, and the plague in medieval Europe (its spread, responses to it and its consequences). We then move on to consider industrialization, urbanization and the rise of scientific medicine, asking whether urbanization created cities of filth and how these developments influenced science and medicine in general, and public health in particular. We then turn to the development of geographical and sociological thinking regarding health, concentrating on the study of suicide by Emile Durkheim and using this as an introduction to seeing variations in health as a combination of individual acts and social facts. We close with an overview of the centuries of change that have been covered and discuss where there has been continuity and where we can see a real break with the past.

Introduction: why take an historical perspective?

The aim of this book is to help you to think about how and why health varies among different groups of people and among different places. One of the best places to begin is in the past. Here we introduce you to some of the ways in which health and illness have been unevenly distributed throughout populations, and how – through research – we can begin to make sense of those inequalities.

We begin by taking an historical perspective. Through looking at past examples we see how patterns of disease have changed over the centuries and that people have had different ways of reacting to and treating illness. People's perceptions of illness and the current global distribution of disease are both very

---

Box 2.1 Social and spatial context

Social context refers to a person's position in society in terms of the social groups they belong to (such as their social class, gender or employment status) and the social roles they perform (e.g. parent, volunteer, employee).

Spatial context refers to a person's geographical location, such as the country, region, town or neighbourhood that they live in, and the features of that place, what that place means to them and the collection of places in which they live during their lives.

---

much products of the past and it is largely through trying to understand the distant and recent past that we attempt to improve our knowledge of health and improve its future distribution.

In taking this historical perspective we also introduce you to thinking about health and illness in sociological and geographical terms. What can sociological and geographical perspectives tell us about health and illness in our society? Putting people in their social and spatial context – in addition to seeing them as individuals – will better help us to understand the causes of illness, and, consequently, how to treat and prevent it (see Box 2.1).

This chapter is not intended as an exhaustive review of the changing patterns of disease in different places over time, nor is it a history of medicine. Instead we use a handful of historical case studies to illustrate how patterns of disease have changed over time, and how in different times and different places there were different causes and consequences of disease. We also begin to introduce sociological and geographical perspectives and show how these can be applied to help us understand how health and illness are intimately connected with the fabric of a society.

The examples considered within this chapter are: traditional medicine, plague in the medieval world, the processes of industrialization and urbanization, and changing rates of suicide. From these examples we can begin to understand the importance of interactions among health, place and society. At the end of the chapter we discuss how an historical view of health and illness shows many changes and developments, but that there are, nonetheless, themes of continuity which emerge.

Potions and prayers: pre-modern societies and traditional medicine

Medicine – the treatment of illness and disease – has not always been practised in the way that it is today. It is only in modern times (see Box 2.2), with the rise of 'science' and the medical profession, that what we now recognize as modern medicine came to develop. In pre-modern societies efforts to heal were dominated not by scientific ideas but by magical or spiritual ways of seeing the world

---

Box 2.2 Types of society

Pre-modern societies	*Hunters and gatherers* – small nomadic groups or tribes which live by hunting, fishing and gathering wild plants to eat.
	Pastoral societies – nomadic people who rear and herd animals, such as sheep, goats and cattle.
	Agrarian societies – people sow and harvest their own crops, and are settled rather than nomadic.
	Traditional societies or civilizations – based on the development of cities, often achieved through conquest. For example, the Roman Empire, the Maya in Mexico, Ancient Egypt.

Modern societies have highly organized divisions of labour brought about through technological changes associated with industrialization and globalization.

(see Box 2.3). Religious beliefs were central to thinking about disease and to approaches to healing it. Prayers or spells were the methods used to attend to illness, often combined with the use of herbal potions – the main form of treatment usually available.

There was not, of course, one single form of medicine practised in all traditional societies; in different times and places there were different traditions. However, what these traditional medical systems have in common is that they tend to be based on religious or spiritual ideas, rather than on a 'rational' basis. In this pre-modern world religion played a central part in all aspects of social life, and this extended to health. Hence, the idea prevailed that disease and illness were caused by supernatural forces – spirits, demons or gods. So an epidemic (or indeed events such as a flood, drought or poor harvest) might have been explained in terms of people's actions making a particular god unhappy and so inciting their wrath.

In order to prevent or cure illness people would appeal to the gods or spirits through prayers, or spells – just as they might appeal for a good harvest. These types of ideas prevailed in Ancient Egypt and were also dominant in the Roman Empire. The Egyptians are thought to have been the first society to have a specialized medical profession but the division between medicine and religion was by no means clear cut; some doctors even came to be regarded as gods them-

---

Box 2.3 Religion and magic

Religion A set of beliefs, symbols and practices based on the idea of the sacred which unites believers into a socio-religious community.

Source: Oxford Dictionary of Sociology.

Magic The influencing of events by the use of potions, chanting or ritual practices. Generally practised by individuals, whereas religion is more organized.

Source: Oxford Dictionary of Sociology.

---

selves. Egyptian medicine combined the use of magic and charms with the use of medicines derived from plants and herbs.

Another traditional medical system is that of Ayurvedic medicine, a system of healing that was developed in India some 3,000–5,000 years ago by Brahmin sages. This was 'holistic' in its approach which means that the individual is considered in their social and environmental context. Ayurvedic medicine focuses on maintaining balance between the three fundamental life energies, rather than on individual symptoms. These three energies, known as the *tridosha*, are: *vata* (ether and air), *pitta* (fire and water) and *kapha* (earth and water). However, this system is individualistic in that two people with the same health problems may need different remedies, because of their energetic constitutions.

Chinese traditional medicine includes the use of many different herbs, which are usually taken in the form of a soup or tea. The philosophy behind this form of medicine is that 'man' lives between heaven and earth, and forms his own universe. There are two forms of energy: material of living things belongs to the '*ying*', which is the female, passive and receding aspect of nature; while functions of living things belong to the '*yang*', the masculine, active and advancing aspect. In order to cure illness, harmony needs to be restored among the five basic elements of earth, fire, water, wood and metal. Such balance could be restored by the use of acupuncture, which controls the flow of energy in the body. Chinese medicine, especially acupuncture, is increasingly popular today in countries all over the world (Figure 2.1).

Looking at another time and place, the Ancient Greeks had a dualistic medical system. On the one hand they believed that there were supernatural causes for illness, but on the other hand they also thought it important to study the symptoms and stages of illness carefully. Two important figures in Greek medicine were Asclepius, the god of healing, and the doctor Hippocrates who lived around 500BC. It is thought that it was Hippocrates who devised the notion that all things were made of four humours – blood, phlegm, black bile and yellow bile – and that illness was related to the loss of balance between

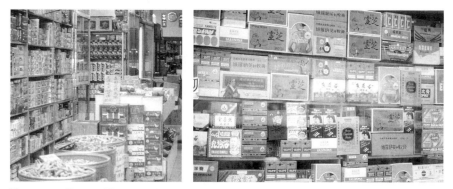

Figure 2.1 Shops selling traditional Chinese medicines and herbs can now be found all over the world.

Source: Photographs by Mary Shaw.

11

them. In Greece and beyond this idea prevailed for two millennia, until the fifteenth century AD.

Hippocrates is still considered to be the father of medicine and he believed that disease had natural causes and that rational methods were needed for cures.

Box 2.4 The Hippocratic Oath – first written 400BC

I SWEAR by Apollo the physician, and Aesculapius, and Health, and All-heal, and all the gods and goddesses, that, according to my ability and judgment, I will keep this Oath and this stipulation to reckon him who taught me this Art equally dear to me as my parents, to share my substance with him, and relieve his necessities if required; to look upon his offspring in the same footing as my own brothers, and to teach them this art, if they shall wish to learn it, without fee or stipulation; and that by precept, lecture, and every other mode of instruction, I will impart a knowledge of the Art to my own sons, and those of my teachers, and to disciples bound by a stipulation and oath according to the law of medicine, but to none others. I will follow that system of regimen which, according to my ability and judgment, I consider for the benefit of my patients, and abstain from whatever is deleterious and mischievous. I will give no deadly medicine to any one if asked, nor suggest any such counsel; and in like manner I will not give to a woman a pessary to produce abortion. With purity and with holiness I will pass my life and practice my Art. I will not cut persons labouring under the stone, but will leave this to be done by men who are practitioners of this work. Into whatever houses I enter, I will go into them for the benefit of the sick, and will abstain from every voluntary act of mischief and corruption; and, further from the seduction of females or males, of freemen and slaves. Whatever, in connection with my professional practice or not, in connection with it, I see or hear, in the life of men, which ought not to be spoken of abroad, I will not divulge, as reckoning that all such should be kept secret. While I continue to keep this Oath unviolated, may it be granted to me to enjoy life and the practice of the art, respected by all men, in all times! But should I trespass and violate this Oath, may the reverse be my lot!

Source: Hippocrates, *Works*, trans. Francis Adams (New York; Loeb) vol. I, 299–301.

The Modern Oath of Hippocrates
This is the version currently approved by the *American Medical Association*:

You do solemnly swear, each by whatever he or she holds most sacred:

- That you will be loyal to the Profession of Medicine and just and generous to its members.
- That you will lead your lives and practice your art in uprightness and honour.
- That into whatsoever house you shall enter, it shall be for the good of the sick to the utmost of your power, your holding yourselves far aloof from wrong, from corruption, from the tempting of others to vice.
- That you will exercise your art solely for the cure of your patients, and will give no drug, perform no operation, for a criminal purpose, even if solicited, far less suggest it.
- That whatsoever you shall see or hear of the lives of men or women which is not fitting to be spoken, you will keep inviolably secret.
- These things do you swear. Let each bow the head in sign of acquiescence. And now, if you will be true to this, your oath, may prosperity and good repute be ever yours; the opposite, if you shall prove yourselves forsworn.

What has been taken out of, and added to, the original version?

He thus based his medicine on observation and reasoning. Hippocrates also had a very strong ethical code and doctors today still swear to the Hippocratic Oath. The original and a current form of the oath are shown in Box 2.4. It is worth noting how the oath has been changed.

Each of these traditional forms of medicine, or medical systems, is embedded in a particular way of seeing the world – a philosophical or ideological framework. There is also a philosophy or ideological framework behind modern western medicine, which we shall come to later in the chapter. It is perhaps easier to recognize ideologies in societies other than your own, because of the very nature of an ideology. Part of the glue that holds society together is the belief that its own particular collective way of viewing the world, its ideology, is *the* way of seeing the world and not simply one of many possible options.

A good way to begin to appreciate that there are very different ways of viewing the world – depending on who you are and where and when you are looking – is to consider the contradictions and contested truths within your own society. If you visit a typical bookshop in a western city you will find they tend to contain many 'self-help' guides to health and well-being. Although modern medicine is the dominant form of health care, people's trust of the conventional medical professions can wax and wane and so people often seek out alternatives. One of the reactions that modern medicine has to this is to incorporate some alternative methods of healing within its fold (see Box 2.5).

Box 2.5 Traditional medicine today

The traditional medical systems are no longer the dominant forms of medicine used in developed societies, but they have not been completely lost. Instead we now refer to them as 'alternative' or 'complementary' forms of medicine. Complementary medicine is becoming increasingly popular in Europe and North America. Some commonly used forms are: acupuncture, aromatherapy, chiropractice, herbal medicine, homeopathy, hypnotherapy, osteopathy, reflexology and yoga. Some medical schools have a complementary medicine component as part of their curriculum.

Percentage of the public reporting use of any form of complementary medicine, *c.* 1990

Country	People reporting use (%)
France	49
Germany	46
USA	34
Belgium	31
UK	26
Sweden	25
Denmark	23
Netherlands	20

Source: adapted from Fisher, P. and Ward, A. (1994). © BMJ Publishing Group

---

In this section we have taken a brief look at some different forms of traditional medicine which originated in very different parts of the pre-modern world. What each of these varied medical systems has in common is that their way of treating illness was a product of their worldview or ideology, and closely connected with spiritual and religious beliefs. In the western world today we have what some might call a 'post-modern' perspective, involving an eclectic mixture of medical systems – we might use Chinese herbal medicine to treat a chronic skin condition, or visit a chiropractor for back pain, but opt for modern medicine for the treatment of a broken leg. We have the ideological freedom (if we have the financial resources) to pick and choose a medical system to treat particular health problems. Nonetheless, despite this pluralism, modern medicine is still the dominant medical system in the West. Before we go on to consider in more detail the context of the development of modern medicine, however, we take a look at the spread of plague through medieval Europe. This is a prime historical example of the intricate connections between disease, place and society.

Rats and fleas: plague in medieval Europe

Box 2.6 The spread of disease

Epidemic A sudden outbreak of a disease that spreads rapidly through a population, affecting large numbers of people. The most common epidemic in western countries is now influenza.

Pandemic An epidemic so widely spread that many people in different countries are affected. AIDS is an example of a pandemic.

Endemic When a disease is constantly found in a particular group of people or in a particular area. Malaria is endemic in much of Africa.

The spread of plague

The plague that ravaged the medieval world, or the Black Death as it later came to be known, is arguably the most mighty example of a *pandemic*. From it we can discover how a biological disease is interwoven with not only the social and the spatial but also environmental factors. The plague was not a new disease; it had always existed among wild rats in certain parts of the world but rarely came into contact with humans. Particular environmental and social conditions led to its tumultuous diffusion through the medieval world (see Box 2.6).

The spread of the plague between 1346 and 1350 is thought to have been precipitated by particular environmental conditions – perhaps floods or earthquakes – which led to these wild rats seeking new food sources and hence coming into close contact with human populations in Central Asia. Particularly mild winters at that time also meant that the spread of the disease was not

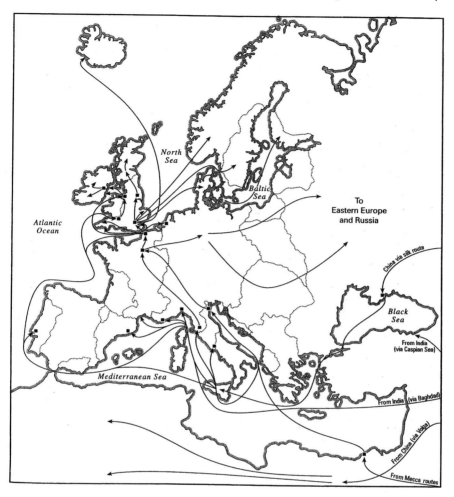

Figure 2.2 Mapping the spread of plague.

abated by harsh weather conditions but spread as quickly in winter as it did in summer. However, rats carried the infection in their blood. They did not pass the disease to humans. Instead they were merely the vehicles for the fleas, and it was when these fed on humans that people became infected.

The first major outbreak of plague originated in China and from there spread along busy caravan routes to India, North Africa (particularly Egypt) and Mesopotamia (now Syria and Iraq) and into the port of Kaffa on the Black Sea (in the Crimea, now a part of Ukraine). From there it spread to Sicily, a busy Italian trading port with connections to the rest of Europe. The map in Figure 2.2 shows the general directions it took.

The trade routes were crucial to the spread of plague, particularly via sea. These routes had connected different societies for centuries but during the

Box 2.7 Symptoms of the plague

All types of plague lead to an unbearable stench carried by sweat, excrement, vomit and breath. Urine can be thick, and black or red.

Bubonic	Pneumonic	Septicaemic
Egg-sized swellings, called buboes, in the lymph glands in the armpits, groin or neck, where the infected flea has bitten	Infection moves into the lungs	Infection enters the bloodstream
Acute, agonizing pain follows with fever, headache and exhaustion	High fever and breathing difficulties	A rash appears; the victim's body literally explodes with the disease
Haemorrhaging under the skin causes purple blotches, often around the waist; the buboes burst	Coughing and sneezing send bacteria into the air and lead to easy spread from person to person	Death can occur within a day
Death results 4–6 days after infection	Victims vomit blood and can choke to death	

medieval period the volume of trade had increased. The rats, and their passenger fleas, travelled aboard ships carrying silks from Asia, and other goods from Italy, through France and Spain, and to Britain. As the sailors and the goods they had transported went ashore, the rats and fleas went with them, spreading the plague. Later the plague travelled on ships to Denmark, Norway and Iceland, and over land across France, Germany, and back into eastern Europe.

As the disease took hold of sea ports, many people fled inland to try to avoid 'the Great Pestilence' as it was known, but in the process they often took the disease with them and passed it on to other people (see Figure 2.3 which portrays people fleeing from London). The better-off were those most likely to have the resources to flee, often leaving behind the impoverished to die first (in Chapter 6 the differential effects of such migrations are considered further). The poor were also at greater risk as the rats preferred their overcrowded dwellings to the more spacious and less penetrable stone-built houses of the more well-to-do. As a greater density of housing meant more rapid transmission, towns had far higher mortality rates than the more dispersed and isolated villages. The highest death rates were in sea and river ports, where the traffic of people, and the flea-carrying rats, was at its greatest (see Box 2.7).

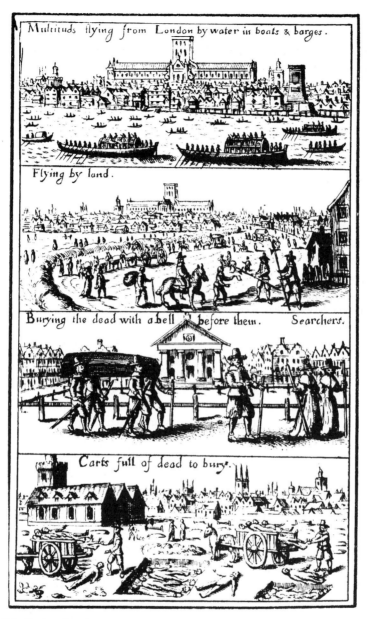

Figure 2.3 Fleeing the plague.

Source: Howe (1972)

Responses to the plague

As well as fleeing and migrating there was a variety of other responses to the plague. People naturally wanted to know what was causing this devastation and theories of explanation proliferated. Some looked to cosmic forces, and saw it as the result of a specific alignment of the planets causing the earth to exude poisonous vapours. Others looked to spiritual sources, seeing it as a scourge sent direct from God in punishment for the sins of humanity.

Others sought to place the blame on particular groups of people – for example, the Jews, who were already generally ill-treated and being expelled from many parts of western Europe. Jewish people were further persecuted as a result of the plague – because they were thought to be agents acting for Satan, accused of poisoning water or of practising witchcraft. Thus we see diseases influencing the structure of society, in this case through repression of particular groups. Half a millennium later we still have a link with this past in that our uncertainty in how best to deal with disease and illness can often have a religious manifestation. The stigmatization of people with AIDS since the 1980s, particularly homosexuals, is an example of how the ideology of religion can sometimes affect the way that we treat people. Ideology or religion can affect how we react to people who have, or whom we think *may* have, a particular illness and how we treat them in both a medical and general sense.

That people were keen to search for the causes of diseases in the fourteenth century, and to place blame, can be related not only to the pervasive spread of the plague, but also to their inability to do anything about it. Medieval medicine had no treatment for the plague, although many different strategies were certainly tried, such as the letting of blood and the burning of aromatic herbs (at least the latter covered the awful stench which exuded from the sufferers). Other responses were more mundane – some contemporary chroniclers reported that the panic produced by the possibility of imminent death led to moral laxity, with people eager to celebrate the comic and profane, and the debauched, while they had the chance. Some also tried the charms and spells of more traditional approaches, and as in many other crises, bells were rung to ward off the disease. Some cities used the more practical method of spatial segregation – quarantine – isolating houses or not allowing ships to dock, but without systematic application this had little effect (see Box 2.8).

Consequences of the plague

In little more than three years the plague had a profound impact upon medieval society. Some describe it as a 'natural disaster', perhaps the greatest ever to affect the population of Europe, but using this term detracts attention from its social and spatial elements. The plague both exacerbated the problems of medieval Europe, created new ones, and solved others (such as the surplus of labour and the shortage of housing).

The demographic impact of the plague was huge – China's population fell from 125 to 90 million and one-third of Europe's population died, perhaps as many as 25 million people. But the reduction in the population was not random. Some areas and some occupations were particularly affected. The busy city of Florence lost up to 75 per cent of its population; clergy and doctors had most contact with the sick and were therefore most likely to get infected themselves.

Box 2.8 Quarantine

Quarantine is the keeping of people or groups in isolation in order to prevent the spread of infectious disease. Leper colonies are an ancient example. Most common was the quarantining of ships in port where there was disease aboard. It was most probably the realization of how the plague was spread geographically that led to this practice. The practice of quarantine to attempt to halt the spread of disease may have later influenced the spatial structure of cities. It may well not be coincidence that the practice of designating social ghettos began in Italian trading cities which were so badly affected by the plague (see Chapter 6 for discussion of the Venice ghetto).

A vastly reduced population led to a shortage of labour – ghost ships drifted with dead crew, fields went untended and half-built cathedrals were left unfinished for many decades. However, a shortage of workers meant that the position of peasants improved, as instead of having to go in search of work, employing landlords now sought them out and offered them better wages and working conditions. Wages soared and the price of land plummeted. The standard of living rose for those who survived as there were more goods to go around. New universities were founded across Europe as a reaction to the loss of the priests who had been society's scholars and teachers.

But while the material conditions of life may have improved as a result of the plague, people lived in constant fear of its return and this is visible in the art of the following period. Ghastly and grisly images of death were common. In spiritual terms, people could not make sense of the epidemic and this led them to be dissatisfied with the Church, sowing the seeds of the decline in its dominance.

Epidemics of plague, on a smaller scale, continued for centuries to come, the last in Britain occurring in 1665. Arguably, no contemporary epidemic has had such a far-reaching influence upon society as did the plague of the medieval world. Yet many of the themes that it illustrates are discernible in other case studies of illnesses that are prevalent today (see Box 2.9).

Box 2.9 Plague in the world today

- Between 1,000 and 3,000 cases occur annually, mostly of the bubonic variety.
- Modern antibiotics can treat the plague, but treatment must be prompt to be effective.
- Modern transport systems mean the disease can now spread extremely quickly.
- When an outbreak of plague occurred in Western India in 1994, 500,000 people fled their homes.
- Plague is one of the diseases that might potentially be used in biological warfare; others include smallpox and anthrax.

Industrialization, urbanization and the rise of scientific medicine

In the section above we discussed some of the many consequences for society of a particular disease epidemic, the plague, one consequence of which was the effect on the labour market. Fewer available labourers meant that they were in greater demand and, for a while at least, their wages and conditions of work improved. In this section we consider a different scenario – the Industrial Revolution in England – and some of the effects that it had on society, health and health care.

The Industrial Revolution, which took place first in England between approximately the mid-eighteenth and the mid-nineteenth centuries, was a time of dramatic change. This was preceded, and overlapped by, the Agricultural Revolution, when new farming technologies (for example, the seed drill), techniques (for instance, crop rotation) and a shift to the cultivation of root crops (such as turnips and potatoes) led to farming being less labour-intensive yet yielding a greater harvest of crops. This meant that more food was produced, and that labour was freed to do other types of work.

The main source of change during the Industrial Revolution was the change in production, from cottage industry where goods were hand-made, to factory production where things were mass-produced by machines. Cotton weaving was the first area to be developed, with the invention of a flying shuttle and

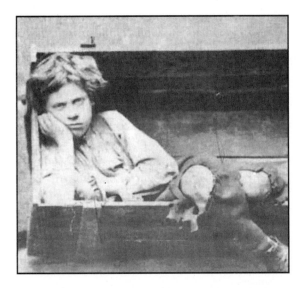

Figure 2.4 A child factory worker of the industrial revolution.

Source: http://www.spartacus.schoolnet.co.uk/IRinspectors.htm

spinning jenny, which speeded up production time considerably. Other important technological developments of the time include steam engines, which were
used as a power source in a variety of contexts, and the railways (following on
from canals) which replaced horse power and greatly increased the capacity for
the movement of goods and people. Many new roads were also built for the distribution of goods within the country; steamships delivered goods to and from
further afield.

While the factory system meant that more goods were available and at
cheaper prices, working conditions in this new industrial environment were
very hard, unpleasant and often harmful. Men, women and children worked
long hours in the factories and they formed the new working class (Figure 2.4).
Pollution of the environment, from factories, mills, mines and the like,
increased massively. In protest at the destruction of the traditional ways of life
and production, workers destroyed many machines, but despite this the process
of industrialization continued.

It is important to note that this development was occurring within a certain
ideological framework – that of *capitalism*. This refers not only to the capitalist
mode of production but also to the power structures that shaped society. Instead
of individuals or small groups of workers labouring independently at home,
people worked in much larger factories. These substantial, purpose-built buildings and the machinery within them required sizeable financial investment,
which was provided by a capitalist owner (in Marxist terms a member of the
'bourgeoisie' – see Box 2.10). The capitalist owned the factory and made a profit
from selling the products of the workers' labour for more than they paid the
workers. It can be argued that the workers were seen by the capitalists as com-
modities, rather than as human beings. In this way wealth was accumulated and
reinvested in other ventures which would accumulate yet more wealth – for the
capitalists.

Urbanization – cities of filth

The changes of the Industrial Revolution were both economic and social. They
also had a huge impact on the human geography of the country. Whereas before
most people had been employed in agriculture and the prevalence of cottage
industries had meant most people lived in rural settings, increasing numbers
of people moved into the cities where the factories were located. The pace of
urbanization was such that the proportion of people living in towns of more
than 5,000 people was 20 per cent in 1801, but by 1851 it was 54 per cent and
by 1911 it was 80 per cent. Thus by the mid-nineteenth century there were
more town than country dwellers for the first time. This rapid congregation of
people in urban areas meant that living conditions were often dirty and filthy –
city living was crowded and insanitary (see Box 2.11). Contagious diseases
thrived in these conditions; cholera was the most virulent, and most feared,
infectious disease (see Chapter 7 for more on cholera).

Box 2.10 Marx and Engels

Karl Marx and his colleague Friedrich Engels sought to explain the changes being wrought on society by the Industrial Revolution, and in particular on social relations and the class struggle, through economics. They developed a materialist view of history, which incorporates the view that social relations are determined by economic relations.

> Modern Industry has converted the little workshop of the patriarchal master into the great factory of the industrial capitalist. Masses of labourers, crowded into the factory, are organised like soldiers. As privates of the industrial army, they are placed under the command of a perfect hierarchy of officers and sergeants. Not only are they slaves of the bourgeois class, and of the bourgeois state; they are daily and hourly enslaved by the machine, by the overlooker, and, above all, in the individual bourgeois manufacturer himself. The more openly this despotism proclaims gain to be its end and aim, the more petty, the more hateful and the more embittering it is.
>
> Karl Marx, *Manifesto of the Communist Party*, Chapter One

Marx's vision was that in the future the capitalist system would be replaced by a society in which there was no longer a ruling capitalist elite dominating the working classes. The means of production would be communally owned, rather than dominated by a few very wealthy and powerful people. Until the fall of Soviet communism, a third of the world's population lived in societies whose governments were based on (various interpretations of) Marx's ideas.

The *rate* of urban growth presented a particular difficulty, and meant that adjustments to accommodate the new urban population were *ad hoc*. Towns were faced with a new set of problems and problems of a huge magnitude. The problems encountered were especially in housing supply and water and sewerage provision. Habits in the towns were not any different from those in the country, but the practices of disposing of waste in the country, where people were more scattered, became a problem when people were packed into towns.

Box 2.11 Letter to *The Times* concerning living conditions in Victorian London

Sur, – May we beg and beseach your proteckshion and power, We are Sur, as it may be, livin in a Wilderness, so far as the rest of London knows anything of us or as the rich and great people care about. We live in muck and filthe. We aint go no priviz, no dust bins, no drains, no water-splies, and no drain or suer in the hole place. ... We all of us suffer, and numbers are ill, and if the Cholera comes Lord help us ...

Preaye Sir come and see us, for we are living like piggs, and it aint faire we should be so ill treeted.

The Times, 5 July 1849

This meant that waste contaminated the water supply, and hence the risk of infection and contagion multiplied. While the better-off middle and upper classes enjoyed better living and working conditions, and were, for example, able to isolate sick children, they too were susceptible to the spread of infectious disease. However, it was the poorest who lived in the worst conditions, and thus suffered the worst health. Figure 2.5 shows that infant mortality rates from diarrhoea and dysentery were highest in the urban industrial centres (such as Birmingham, Liverpool, Manchester and Newcastle).

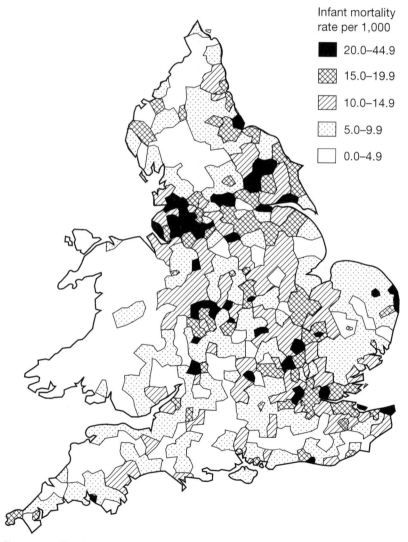

Infant mortality
rate per 1,000

- 20.0–44.9
- 15.0–19.9
- 10.0–14.9
- 5.0–9.9
- 0.0–4.9

Figure 2.5 Diarrhoea and dysentery deaths in infants, England and Wales, 1861–1870.

Source: Woods and Shelton (1997).

Nutrition was also poor in the urban environment. Women particularly suffered from poor nutrition, as even at the best times men would get more of any meat available; women would get the scraps. This had a knock-on effect for the health of babies and children. As well as problems with the *amount* of food that people ate there were also great problems concerning the *quality* of food. Cow's milk, for example, was often kept in filthy conditions – stored in dirty buckets and churns with no lids, and, of course, there was no effective refrigeration. This was particularly important as working women (who for financial reasons often had to work until very late in their pregnancy and very soon after giving birth) were unable to breast-feed their babies. The cow's milk that many children were fed was contaminated. Inadequate excrement removal also led to the contamination of food, via hands and flies.

Lack of adequate nutrition is an important health indicator in itself, but also means that people, especially children, are more prone to infectious diseases. Poor nutritional conditions were also compounded by arduous labour, damp, cold and overcrowded housing and inadequate sanitation. Overcrowding meant spending a lot of time outdoors where children without adequate clothing would catch cold. Indoors, living in cramped conditions, often with many

---

Box 2.12 The physical deterioration of the textile workers

Any man who has stood at twelve o'clock at the single narrow door-way, which serves as the place of exit for the hands employed in the great cotton-mills, must acknowledge, that an uglier set of men and women, of boys and girls, taking them in the mass, it would be impossible to congregate in a smaller compass. Their complexion is sallow and pallid – with a peculiar flatness of feature, caused by the want of a proper quantity of adipose substance to cushion out the cheeks. Their stature low – the average height of four hundred men, measured at different times, and different places, being five feet six inches. Their limbs slender, and playing badly and ungracefully. A very general bowing of the legs. Great numbers of girls and women walking lamely or awkwardly, with raised chests and spinal flexures. Nearly all have flat feet, accompanied with a down-tread, differing very widely from the elasticity of action in the foot and ankle, attendant upon perfect formation. Hair thin and straight – many of the men having but little beard, and that in patches of a few hairs, much resembling its growth among the red men of America. A spiritless and dejected air, a sprawling and wide action of the legs, and an appearance, taken as a whole, giving the world but 'little assurance of a man,' or if so, 'most sadly cheated of his fair proportions …'

Factory labour is a species of work, in some respects singularly unfitted for children. Cooped up in a heated atmosphere, debarred the necessary exercise, remaining in one position for a series of hours, one set or system of muscles alone called into activity, it cannot be wondered at – that its effects are injurious to the physical growth of a child. Where the bony system is still imperfect, the vertical position it is compelled to retain, influences its direction; the spinal column bends beneath the weight of the head, bulges out laterally, or is dragged forward by the weight of the parts composing the chest, the pelvis yields beneath the opposing pressure downwards, and the resistance given by the thigh-bones; its capacity is lessened, sometimes more and sometimes less; the legs curve, and the whole body loses height, in consequence of this general yielding and bending of its parts.

P. Gaskell (1833), pp. 161–2, 202–3.

people sharing a single room and one bed, meant that diseases were easily spread from person to person. It was infants and children who bore the brunt of these conditions. Infant and child mortality was for the large part responsible for average life expectancy in England and Wales being 40 for men and 42 for women in 1841, when proper records were first made (ONS, 1998). Dramatic decreases in infant and child mortality in the late nineteenth century and through the twentieth century, rather than improvements in life expectancy at older ages, were mainly responsible for the greater total life expectancy we now enjoy.

Thus the living and working conditions (see Box 2.12) of the expanding towns of the Industrial Revolution were seen by many as inevitably leading to disease and death; there was no doubt that industrialisation was bad for health, and the health of the population was a constant concern.

Developments in science and medicine

Box 2.13 The Enlightenment

The Enlightenment occurred throughout the eighteenth century and refers to the turn away from the dominant religious paradigm and folk traditions towards the use of reason. Many believed that the world could be changed, indeed vastly improved, by the pursuit of reason and truth. Doctors, and the pursuit of scientific and medical knowledge, were a key part of this change. Hospitals became the centre of the development of medical knowledge.

In the eighteenth and nineteenth centuries, as well as advances in production and the process of urbanization, there were at the same time many developments in science and in medicine (see Box 2.13). These included innovations such as vaccinations, X-rays and pasteurization. As noted above, ideas about medicine had previously been dominated by religious or spiritual notions. But during this time there was a radical shift away from spiritual ideologies towards scientific medicine or 'biomedicine'. Two ideas are intricately connected with the development of biomedicine. The first is the Cartesian Revolution, which taught that mind and body were separate. The second is the idea that each disease has its own specific aetiology, or cause, which is biological in origin. The body was viewed in a very physical way; there was no space for broader notions of psychological, or indeed social, well-being (contrast this to the World Health Organization definition of health in Box 2.14). Germ theory was developed at this time, which was the idea that each disease has a single specific cause. The

---

Box 2.14 A definition of health

A complete sense of physical, mental and social well-being and not merely the absence of disease.

Source: WHO (1947).

Box 2.15 Medicalization

Medicalization started during the nineteenth century when greater numbers of doctors were trained and they became more and more powerful in influencing areas of life beyond the practice of medicine. Doctors and medicine became increasingly pervasive in modern life as areas of life became increasingly subject to the medical gaze, e.g. birth and death, drug use and even gambling. Many feminists see the medicalization of pregnancy and childbirth as taking control away from women.

---

focus of the new scientific medicine was thus very much on the level of the cell and the micro-organisms producing disease, rather than on the person as a whole or their broader environment or community.

Advocates of scientific medicine, or biomedicine, like to think of themselves as objective and value-free (as part of the Enlightenment search for truth). Under this paradigm, facts are collected by the scientific method (using controlled experiments). However, a sociological perspective argues that we can never by wholly value-free, rather our activities are always in the context of, and influenced by, the society in which we live, and by its values.

Whether we consider it to be value-free or value-laden, scientific medicine came to be the dominant medical system and, as a group of people, doctors became very powerful (see Box 2.15). The number of medical practitioners grew, and they formed powerful professional organizations. There was also much expansion of hospitals, which grew in number and were the centre of medical education, where doctors learnt by clinical example. We should note, however, that the establishment of the medical profession was a male preserve. Until the eighteenth century healing had been predominantly women's work, but in the eighteenth and nineteenth centuries women were increasingly excluded from practising medicine. Not until 1875 were women permitted to attend medical school (see Box 2.16). Feminists argue that in this way the development of scientific medicine was value-laden, in that it incorporated a patriarchal ideology that excluded women and gave power and prestige to men.

Box 2.16 Elizabeth Blackwell (1821–1910)

Elizabeth Blackwell was the first woman to graduate from medical school (Geneva Medical College in New York State, United States) in the modern era (in 1849). However, her admittance led to the college formally closing entry for woman and many other medical schools also had rules to exclude women. The University of Zurich was the first to formally allow women to study there in the 1860s. The London School of Medicine for Women was opened in London in 1874, but it was many years before women were allowed access to the most prestigious schools of medicine. Women were not permitted to study medicine at Harvard University until 1947.

Public health

Scientific medicine has become so dominant in ideological terms that we tend to view it uncritically and see it as a positive factor, and as *the* explanation for improved health and life expectancy over recent centuries. Until the early part of the twentieth century the drugs and surgical techniques used by the medical profession were for the most part ineffective. We must therefore ask the crucial question: to what extent do improvements in medical treatment account for the substantial increases in life expectancy that we (in the industrial world) have enjoyed over the past 150 years?

Alongside developments in the very individualistic approach of scientific medicine there were many in the Victorian era who were passionately concerned with the effect of squalid living and working conditions on the health of the population, and in particular the poor, and in alleviating those conditions. It was this concern with the connection of broader social and environmental conditions that led to the establishment of, and improvements in, public health (see Box 2.17).

Box 2.17 Public health

Public health is concerned with assessing the needs and trends on health and disease of populations as distinct from individuals. Formerly known as community or social medicine.

Source: Oxford Concise Medical Dictionary.

McKeown (1976) considered the role of medicine in producing the decline in mortality seen towards the end of the nineteenth century and noted that declines in many diseases – such as tuberculosis, whooping cough, cholera and scarlet fever – preceded the availability of effective medical treatment. However, the case of smallpox McKeown sees as an exception, where medical intervention through vaccination seems to be responsible for the subsequent decline in mortality. For other diseases, McKeown sees improvements in nutrition, linked to a rise in real wages, as the determining factor in improving population health. Better food in terms of quantity (afforded by improved wages) and quality (in terms of regulations concerning adulteration and the range of foods available) would have been particularly beneficial to the health of babies and children. Others point to improvements in the water supply (see Box 2.18), and the building of a system for the removal of sewage and improvements in housing conditions, as probable key factors in the improvement of the health of the public. The public health reforms of the Victorian era were thus a key ingredient to improving life expectancy in countries such as England.

Public health, it must be noted, is very much linked to the ideology of the state, as decisions have to made about which health issues to use resources to act upon, and which to leave alone. Many Victorians were concerned with public health because they saw a need for a healthy workforce, and for fit men to be in the armed forces – the needs of the economy, and of the state, were foremost in their concerns. We could even say that public health for the Victorians took the

Box 2.18 The River Thames – would you want to drink it?

The Thames was used as a sewer for human and animal excrement, as well as a dumping ground for the waste from various industries – such as the tanning of leather or the dyeing of materials. Even offal from slaughterhouses found its way into the river. As a result the river was a dark stinking mess, often covered in a frothy scum. This was also the water that Londoners drank.

Observations on the Filth of the Thames, contained in a letter addressed to the Editor of *The Times* Newspaper, by Professor Faraday

SIR,

I traversed this day by steam-boat the space between London and Hungerford Bridges between half-past one and two o'clock; it was low water, and I think the tide must have been near the turn. The appearance and the smell of the water forced themselves at once on my attention. The whole of the river was an opaque pale brown fluid. In order to test the degree of opacity, I tore up some white cards into pieces, moistened them so as to make them sink easily below the surface, and then dropped some of these pieces into the water at every pier the boat came to; before they had sunk an inch below the surface they were indistinguishable, though the sun shone brightly at the time; and when the pieces fell edgeways the lower part was hidden from sight before the upper part was under water. This happened at St. Paul's Wharf, Blackfriars Bridge, Temple Wharf, Southwark Bridge, and Hungerford; and I have no doubt would have occurred further up and down the river. Near the bridges the feculence rolled up in clouds so dense that they were visible at the surface, even in water of this kind.

The smell was very bad, and common to the whole of the water; it was the same as that which now comes up from the gully-holes in the streets; the whole river was for the time a real sewer. Having just returned from out of the country air, I was, perhaps, more affected by it than others; but I do not think I could have gone on to Lambeth or Chelsea, and I was glad to enter the streets for an atmosphere which, except near the sink-holes, I found much sweeter than that on the river.

I have thought it a duty to record these facts, that they may be brought to the attention of those who exercise power or have responsibility in relation to the condition of our river; there is nothing figurative in the words I have employed, or any approach to exaggeration; they are the simple truth. If there be sufficient authority to remove a putrescent pond from the neighbourhood of a few simple dwellings, surely the river which flows for so many miles through London ought not to be allowed to become a fermenting sewer. The condition in which I saw the Thames may perhaps be considered as exceptional, but it ought to be an impossible state, instead of which I fear it is rapidly becoming the general condition. If we neglect this subject, we cannot expect to do so with impunity; nor ought we to be surprised if, ere many years are over, a hot season give us sad proof of the folly of our carelessness.

I am, Sir,
Your obedient servant,
M. FARADAY.
Royal Institution, July 7, 1855

Source: The Times Newspaper, London, 7 July 1855.

form of a moral crusade – epidemics were not seen as punishments from God, but as a sign of 'man's' neglect of society; the physical improvement of the population was seen as a necessary basis for moral and intellectual improvement.

Whereas public health reforms in Victorian society were aimed at environmental issues such as sanitation, the focus of current interventions is aimed more towards the prevention of disease associated with behavioural factors. This shift is partly connected with changes in the major causes of death – away from infectious diseases towards chronic diseases such as heart disease and cancer – but the shift is also ideological. In the contemporary context there are very strong political and economic reasons why smoking, which has been proven to be extremely bad for health in a number of ways, is *not* banned, not least of all the consideration of the amount of tax revenue tobacco sales bring. The banning of smoking has many potential consequences – the improvement of health and less use of health services, but extended life expectancy would mean more old-age pensions to pay. Public health measures to reduce smoking tend to be focused at the individual rather than the societal level, thus avoiding major changes to structural arrangements, and in the process effectively 'blaming the individual'.

In this section, then, we have considered the case of the Industrial Revolution in England, and the consequences of this and other associated developments on the health of the population. The health of particular groups in society – the poor and labouring classes – was particularly affected, and poor health was most apparent in certain areas – the new urban industrial centres. We have also considered developments in the medical arena and the establishment of the (male) medical profession and the role of public health reforms. A key theme of this section has been the role of dominant ideologies in affecting both the organization of society and the health of a population. In the next section we take a closer look at the development of a sociological perspective.

Suicide: an individual act or a social fact?

In this section we consider the case of suicide, and we also learn how the discipline of sociology developed, and what constitutes a sociological perspective. We have already introduced the point of view of Friedrich Engels and Karl Marx and briefly touched on how their perspective on society came to be organized as it was. They were directly influenced by the poor health of Victorian Britain described above, which they witnessed first hand. What did other sociologists have to say on the subject of the sociology of health?

There are many different conditions that can lead to death, but one that is found in all societies and has been apparent throughout history, is self-inflicted death, or suicide. Suicide stands out as significantly different from other causes of death and can be seen as a most individual act. For their own personal reason, someone chooses to die, as well as how they will die. In this respect it seems to be the ultimately individual way to die. However, closer study reveals that there are social as well as geographical patterns to suicide. Where you live and who you are can affect your likelihood of dying from this most personal cause of death. The study of suicide is linked with the early development of sociology.

Durkheim and the development of sociology

In the early nineteenth century the scientific approach which had been developed in order to study the natural world also came to be applied to understanding society. The great social changes that had followed the French Revolution of 1789 and the English Industrial Revolution as well as the legacy of the Enlightenment, which emphasized the application of reason and rationality and the notion of progress, meant that there was a greater impetus to understand and scrutinize the social world. The new discipline of sociology sought to understand why society was structured in the way it was, and how and why change came about.

Auguste Comte, who coined the word 'sociology', believed that by collecting scientific evidence, a knowledge of society and the way that it worked could be built up. Emile Durkheim took this further and saw the subject matter of sociology as 'social facts'. He saw social facts as things that were external to individuals, characteristics of societies rather than of individual people. For instance, a person's chances of succeeding in education can be seen as depending more on the society they live in than on themselves (Durkheim was one of the first to write on the theory of equality of opportunity in education).

Sociologists see social entities existing 'over and above' individuals and consider that these entities persist over time, as the individuals in any place change and are replaced by a new generation – social facts continue. For instance, the students and staff of a university may change over time, but the organizational structure remains essentially the same (the structure of the academic year, the setting of assignments and examinations, graduation ceremonies) and the activities of the students, both official and unofficial, persist (for example, rag week or end of term parties).

Social entities have the effect of placing constraints on the way people act. Examples of such restraints are laws which are established by the authority of the state (such as laws that relate to the use of roads), or customs (such as the custom of letting people pull into a queue of traffic). These are not only imposed on the individual, formally or informally, but are internalized by individuals (traffic is, for the main part, self-regulated) – individuals feel a moral obligation to stick to the rules. In this sense society is both beyond and within individuals. Social entities are also greater than the sum of their constituent parts – a football team, for example, is much more than the players that make it up (who change over time); the team itself has characteristics and an identity (see Box 2.19).

In thinking about how social order was maintained Durkheim also gave much consideration to the relationship between the individual and society. He theorized that people as individuals have unlimited desires but that these are controlled by regulative social forces which exert a pressure on people to behave

---

Box 2.19 Some key sociological issues and terms

Social order How and why is social order maintained? What holds societies together? Are they held together by shared values, or is conflict constrained by powerful groups controlling the weak?

Social structure The practices and institutions that can be found in a society and that structure the organization of social life. These can be institutions in the literal sense, such as schools or hospitals, or symbolic, such as the 'institution' of the family.

The state A set of institutions which has the authority to govern society.

Culture Everything in society that is learnt socially rather than transmitted biologically.

Rituals A repeated behaviour performed at a particular time, usually involving the use of symbols (something that represents something else). For instance, religious rituals, such as the giving of communion in some parts of the Christian church, where the wafer represents the body of Christ; an example of a secular ritual is the parading of a team mascot (a symbol) before a football match.

Norms The informal rules of society which indicate the shared expectations of how people should behave.

(Social) theory An explanation of why the social world (or part of it) is the way it is, drawing on various concepts.

---

in a certain way. However, when these forces break down, and individuals are left to their own devices, then a condition of *anomie* prevails and behaviour is no longer regulated by common norms.

But why did Durkheim choose to look at suicide? Durkheim looked at suicide as a social fact rather than an individual act. He observed that over time different places tend to have similar suicide rates each year, even though each year completely different individuals choose to take their own lives. The suicide rate is a social fact – the rate being distinct from the individual acts that make it. The rate belongs to society. He thus saw the suicide rate as something *sui generis* – in itself – to be explained.

Figure 2.6 shows the suicide rates per million of the population for various parts of Europe over three time periods between 1866 and 1878. What is striking about the graph is that there are large differences in the suicide rates of the different places, but also that the rates are fairly stable over time – the rate in Saxony (now part of Germany) is consistently high whereas in Italy it is consistently low. As Durkheim himself noted (1999 edition, page 46):

> If, instead of seeing in them separate occurrences, unrelated and to be separately studied, the suicides committed in a given society during a given period of time are taken as a whole, it appears that this total is not simply a sum of independent units, a collective total, but is itself a new fact *sui generis*, with its own unity, individuality and consequently its own nature – a nature, futhermore, dominantly social. Indeed, provided too long a period is not considered, the statistics for one and the same society are almost invariable ...

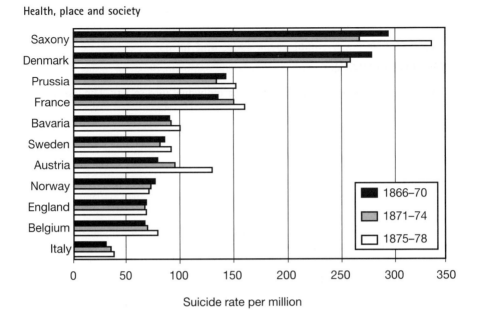

Figure 2.6 Suicide in Europe, 1866–78.

Source: Drawn from data in Durkheim (1999).

In his book, Durkheim presents a systematic analysis of these rates, amalgamating a number of different sources of data which had never before been compared. He first considered a variety of possible explanations – such as mental alienation, characteristics of 'race', hereditary factors, climate and temperature. However, his analysis revealed that suicide rates were instead related to social phenomena – the family, political, economic and religious structures in society. The rate of suicide can therefore only be understood within the social structure within which it occurs.

Durkheim was particularly interested in how the integration of individuals within society was related to suicide rates, and lack of integration might lead to anomie. Integration can be achieved through a variety of means, including family support and religious affiliation, or through work. He noted that when a society is strongly integrated, with strong social bonds and a high degree of social cohesion, suicide rates are low, since during hard times people are cushioned by those bonds and thus less likely to resort to extreme responses such as suicide. Low levels of social integration on the other hand mean that in difficult times people may not have support mechanisms and that they may resort to individualistic solutions to problems. However, integration is not always a good thing. People can become over-integrated into social norms, and they can effectively be 'brainwashed' into sacrificing their individual life for the sake of the goals of society. Durkheim related these different levels of integration to different types of suicide (see Box 2.20).

> **Box 2.20 Durkheim's types of suicide – according to the relationship of the actor to society**
>
> **Egoistic suicide** Lack of integration of the individual into society. The less individuals are integrated into the wider social fabric, the more vulnerable they are to suicide. This can refer to the societal level, or to family integration. For example, someone who lives alone and has few social or family contacts.
>
> **Altruistic suicide (opposite to egoistic)** When the individual is overly integrated into social regulations so that they take their life when norms demand, e.g. Hindu widows committing suicide on the funeral pyres of their husbands; or the Japanese tradition of Hara-kiri.
>
> **Anomic suicide** When the normative regulations guiding people are relaxed, when collective conscience weakens. Particularly refers to the way that people are affected by the economic context of society. For example, suicide occurring after suddenly becoming wealthy or impoverished.

Durkheim explained the differential rates of different groups of people and in different places using these concepts. For example, he explained the higher rates of suicide found in Protestant populations compared with Catholic populations as produced by the greater degree of social integration of the Catholics (and to Catholic teaching). Protestantism, on the other hand, encourages greater independence and autonomy, and greater freedom to individual thought. Durkheim also relates the low rates of suicide among Jews to high levels of group solidarity, brought about in part by their forced exclusion by other social groups leading to a strong sense of group identity and unity.

At the micro-level of the family (see Box 2.21), Durkheim uses the concept of social integration to explain the lower suicide rates of married people compared with the unmarried, although the 'protective' effect is generally greater for men than for women. He attributes this to the influence of the domestic environment, and having more to do with family/children than to do with partnership *per se*. It is also the case that larger families have lower suicide rates. Why? Suicide rates are low when collective sentiments are strong; the more people in a family unit to reinforce those sentiments, the stronger the integration.

Durkheim's work is important to developing a sociological viewpoint as it showed the importance of social factors in a phenomenon that is apparently completely individual – suicide rates can be explained by reference to the social structure. Durkheim thus showed that society (like a football team) is more than the sum of its constituent parts. As well as his approach and conceptualization, his work is also important in the way he approached the problem to be unravelled – he tackled the data in a systematic and rigorous manner. This was at a time not only before computing, but when the methods of statistics were in their infancy. Another important legacy of this work is that it laid foundations for an alternative to the medical model.

Box 2.21 Macro and micro

Macro refers to the wider structures of society and global and historical changes on a large scale.

Micro refers to social processes on a smaller scale, where interaction takes place, meanings are constructed and negotiated.

A number of criticisms have been directed at Durkheim's work, particularly regarding the problem of collecting data about suicide. For example, different societies may define suicide in different ways, and some groups may be reluctant to report suicides and more likely to report deaths as accidental, thus suppressing the true rate. There are also broader issues with the application of the scientific method to studying the social world, not least the fact that the subjects, unlike the particles in physics or compounds in chemistry, are conscious beings and not docile objects.

However, Durkheim's work on suicide continues to influence its study, and there is evidence that the concepts he developed are still relevant today. A recent study, for example, found that anomie still predicts suicide rates well. This ecological study looked at suicide rates at the constituency level in England and Wales (Whitley *et al.*, 1999) and found that anomie (which they refer to as 'social fragmentation') predicted suicide more strongly than did measures of poverty (Chapter 3 includes a more detailed description of this research). The measure of social fragmentation they used included the number of people

---

Box 2.22 The Samaritans

A nationwide (British) charity, founded in 1953, which exists to provide confidential emotional support to any person, irrespective of race, creed, age or status, who is suicidal or despairing. They also aim to increase public awareness of issues around suicide and depression.

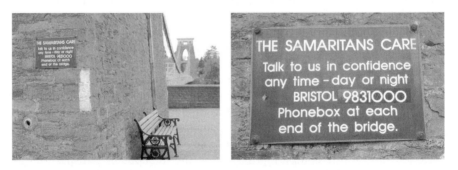

Figure 2.7 Samaritans sign at the Clifton suspension bridge, Bristol.

Source: Photographs by Mary Shaw.

renting their homes, single person households (under the age of 65), mobility in the previous year and the proportion of unmarried people – one of the indicators used by Durkheim. At the end of the twentieth century the importance of social integration and social support in determining suicide rates can still be seen (see Box 2.22).

Conclusion

Centuries of change

In this chapter we have considered various case studies which show how health, place and society interact. Sociological and geographical perspectives can help us to unpick and understand these connections; in the next chapter we look more closely at sociological and geographical methods that we can apply in this context.

We began by looking at the spread of the plague in the early modern era; we also considered the spread of infectious diseases under the very different conditions of the Industrial Revolution. The Industrial Revolution wrought many far-reaching changes upon society, changing the nature of work, conditions of living and the structure of social relations. Patterns of health, and of health care, were also dramatically altered. In advanced industrial societies the main causes of death are no longer infectious diseases, but are instead chronic non-infectious diseases. The pattern of disease in society is related to the way that society lives and how it is organized, such as patterns of trade, types of housing, household structure and, of course, basic determinants such as access to resources like water. Even causes of death that seem to be completely individual, such as suicide, are affected by social conditions and social processes.

Through these various case studies we have also seen how there are different approaches to medicine and health care, and how these have developed. In western societies, the role of religion, both in terms of medicine and more generally, has declined – a process known as secularization. In its place scientific medicine, sometimes referred to as biomedicine, has come to dominate the medical and health-care system. This has now become such a dominant ideology – a way of seeing the world – in which many areas of life which were not previously considered to be medical concerns have been medicalized.

Themes of continuity

Despite the many changes that we can observe through considering these historical examples, there are also many themes of continuity. The role of ideology has been apparent throughout, whether this is a 'religious' or 'scientific' way of viewing the world. Despite the claims of scientific medicine that it is (or at least aims to be) objective and value-free, a sociological perspective allows us to recognize that our values constantly pervade our actions and become entrenched in the social structures we build. Scientific medicine, for example, has hardly been value-free in terms of its treatment, in the broadest sense, of women. Women are now able to join the medical profession from which they were initially excluded, yet they continue to face many barriers to career progression and are concentrated in the lower-paid and less prestigious jobs. Meanwhile, as the subjects of medicine, women have often been trivialized, and many areas of their lives medicalized. It should also be noted that most health care has historically been, and is still, provided by women, as they make up the majority of carers in the formal (as nurses) and informal (as carers at home) sectors.

In the same way that medicine and health care are value-laden, this chapter and this book as a whole are also affected by values. As authors, what we write is influenced by the society from which we originate (and others we have experienced) and by the knowledge and experiences that we have accrued (see Figure 1.1). Our 'geographical' background, for example, is obvious in that this is a very Anglo-centric chapter (this is something that we attempt to redress somewhat in later chapters). This perspective, and other values that we hold, has affected the topics and themes that we selected, and the points we have chosen to highlight. What we have included is what we think is important. Throughout this book we encourage you to be aware of this and to develop critical thinking through your awareness.

Another source of continuity is that while a scientific approach, to medicine and other areas of life, has come to dominate western society, other approaches to the medical model have proliferated in recent years. Greater criticism of and lack of trust in western medicine have led many people to turn to alternative or traditional forms of medicine, as we noted above. Many people prefer the holistic approach that these different medical systems incorporate.

In addition to this there are still many 'non-scientific' aspects to the way we respond to and treat disease. We still have social responses to ill-health. Certain illnesses, and certain groups of people, are still stigmatized and, in extreme cases, refused treatment or even persecuted; others are seen as 'innocent victims'. Contrast, for example, the way that western society has responded to homosexuals and injecting drug users with HIV/AIDS, compared with those haemophiliacs who became infected through blood transfusions.

It is not just in the field of ideology or values that we can see continuities with the past, there are also continuities of an empirical nature – in the measurable patterns of health in terms of its social and spatial distribution. While for industrialized western nations infectious diseases are no longer the main cause of mortality, in the poorer countries of the world these continue to be predominant. While living and working conditions clearly differ in many ways from the early days of the Industrial Revolution in England, matters of food and water supply, housing and the organization of labour still impact upon health. In particular, many of the health hazards facing Victorian working-class men and women (and their children) are very similar to those faced in the 'developing' world today.

Despite many changes in the social world, there are some enduring themes in the study of health, place and society about which we can compare empirical

---

Box 2.23 Infant mortality over a century: absolute falls, but relative differences remain

In England and Wales in 1891–95 infant mortality rates were 151 per 1000; in 1991–95 the rate was 6 per 1000.

ONS (1998)

… in London in 1891, the infant death rate in a poor and crowded district such as the Strand was approximately double that of a solidly middle-class area such as Plumstead. …To be born to poor parents at the beginning of the century meant that one was twice as likely to die before reaching one's first birthday.

Wohl (1983), pp. 39–41

The richer the family and community a child is born into, the more likely they are to be healthy, even in the first year of life … infant mortality rates are 2.0 times higher for those in the highest mortality [for adults under 65] constituencies compared to the lowest mortality constituencies.

Shaw *et al.* (1999), pp. 16–17

---

evidence. Arguably the central theme is that, then and now, poorer folk have worse life chances than do wealthy folk. Even though the main causes of death have changed, unequal life chances persist. As Box 2.23 indicates, while infant mortality has fallen dramatically in absolute terms, in relative terms social and spatial inequalities persist.

This persistent inequality can be seen in the results of some recent research (Dorling *et al.*, 2000). New technology means that we can revisit old sources of data. In this case we digitized a map of poverty in London at the end of the nineteenth century, which had been assembled by the pioneer social researcher Charles Booth in 1889 (see Booth, 1969). We could then compare this with a map of poverty for London at the end of the twentieth century, this time using the 1991 census of population. What is remarkable about the results is that, by and large, the social and spatial distributions of the wealth/poverty structure of London have remained very similar – rich areas tend to have stayed rich and poor areas remain poor. In addition to this, we are able to see how these two measures of poverty, relate to the current geography of mortality in London. The results show that Booth's measure of social class in London at the end of the nineteenth century is as good as the 1991 census at predicting mortality at the end of the twentieth century. Thus just as the ranking between social groups tends to persist over time, so too can the ranking of places. Despite a century of rapid and far-reaching social change, the medical geography of London is very similar to what it was a century ago many other 'changes' also often turn out to have occurred before (see Figure 2.8).

Thus in considering health, place and society in historical perspective there are themes of both change and continuity; the perspectives of medical geography and medical sociology can help us to unpick and understand those themes.

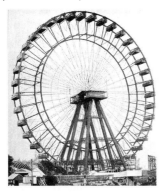 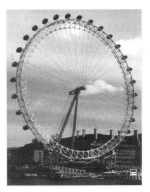

Figure 2.8 Big wheel at Earl's Court (1896) and the London Eye (2000).

Source: Earl's Court from Lewis (1998); London Eye photograph by Mary Shaw.

Further reading

- Defoe, Daniel (1969) *A Journal of the Plague Year: being Observations or Memorials of the most Remarkable Occurrences, as well Publick as Private, which happened in London during the last Great Visitation in 1665.* Oxford University Press: London.

  In this classic book Defoe uses the literary technique of a journal, written by the fictitious saddler Henry Foe, and tells the tale of the plague in London. He uses Bills of Mortality (which were published weekly by each parish) to describe the temporal and geographical spread of the plague. These historical data are accompanied by much descriptive detail, and the historical event comes alive as we read of Foe's struggle to survive and his reflections in conditions where normal day-to-day activities are suspended. It presents not only a description of the extent and spread of the plague but also consideration of the social, economic, religious and philosophical questions raised by the plague. In addition the book is not so much about the individuals affected but about the corporate nature of the plague – how it affected London as a place; it is thus a narrative of the stricken city of London.

- Goffman, Erving (1961) *Asylums: Essays on the Social Situation of Mental Patients and Other Inmates.* Penguin: Harmondsworth.

  During the 1950s Goffman spent much time observing the details of the fabric of social life inside the closed community, or 'total institution', of a mental asylum. A total institution is Goffman's term for a place of residence where a large number of people in a similar situation live together, cut off from the rest of society, in a way of life that is bounded by the formality of rules and regulations. Examples of total institutions include prisons and monasteries. Goffman writes from the point of view of the inmates rather than the staff and through detailed descriptions shows the sense of betrayal and loss of identity that an inmate feels when they enter a new institution, and how they cope and adapt to a new way of life.

- Becker, H., Geer, B., Hughes, E.C. and Strauss, A. (1961) *Boys in White: Student Culture in Medical School.* University of Chicago Press: Chicago.

  This is a classic in medical sociology and reports the results of a study of the University of Kansas Medical School in the 1950s. The title reflects the male domination of the profession at that time and follows the process of how 'boys become medical men'. This process, of becoming a doctor, is a rite of passage: 'A rite of passage is that series of instructions, ceremonies, and ordeals by which those already in a special status initiate neophytes into their charmed circle, by which men turn boys into fellow men, fit to be their own companions and successors.' Using symbolic interactionism as their theoretical framework, the researchers conducted a qualitative, unstructured investigation using overt participant observation to get at the processes through which an individual is made into a doctor.

- Leavitt, Judith Walzer (1996) *Typhoid Mary: Captive to the Public's Health*. Beacon Press: Boston.

  Mary Mallon was born in Ireland in 1869 and emigrated to the United States as a teenager, where she worked as a cook in New York. She was a carrier of typhoid fever, and through her cooking infected 22 people, one of whom died. The authorities reacted by forcibly confining her to live alone in a small bungalow in the grounds of an isolation hospital on North Brother Island. This book tells her story from a number of different perspectives – showing different dimensions of America's response to sickness and sickness control. The story of 'Typhoid Mary' raises many issues, concerning our social and spatial responses to those who pose a threat to the health of the public by carrying or through suffering illness, that are still relevant today.

Suggested activities

- A film to watch: *The Horseman on the Roof* (directed by Jean-Paul Rappeneau) is based on the classic novel by Jean Giono. This is the story of an outbreak of cholera in Provence in 1832. The devastating physical effects of the disease are shown, as well as the responses of society (fear, flight, quarantine).
- Look at how illness and death have been portrayed in the art of different eras, different societies and different artists.
- Find out about health, society and poverty in the area where you live, now and in the past. What has and hasn't changed?

References

Booth, C. (1969, first published 1889) *Life and Labour of the People of London. First Series, Poverty (I) East, Central and South London*. Macmillan and Co. Ltd: London.

Dorling, D., Mitchell, R., Shaw, M., Orford, S. and Davey Smith, G. (2000) The Ghost of Christmas Past: the health effects of poverty in London in 1896 and 1991. *British Medical Journal*, 321: 1547–51.

Durkheim, E. (1999, first published 1897) *Suicide: A Study in Sociology*. Routledge: London.

Fisher, P. and Ward, A. (1994) Medicine in Europe: complementary medicine in Europe. *BMJ*, 309: 107–11.

Gaskell, P. (1833) *The Manufacturing Population of England*. London.

Howe, G.M. (1972) *Man, Environment and Disease in Britain: A Medical Geography of Britain Through the Ages*. David & Charles: Newton Abbot.

Lewis, P. (1998) *London 100 Years Ago: A Photographic Record*. Parkgate Books: London.

Marx, K. and Engels, F. (1998) *The Communist Manifesto: A Modern Edition*. With an introduction by Eric Hobsbawm. Verso: London.

McKeown, T. (1976) *The Modern Rise of Population*. Edward Arnold: London.

Office for National Statistics (1998) *Mortality Statistics: General 1996*. Series DH1 No. 29. The Stationery Office: London.

Shaw, M., Gordon, D., Dorling, D. and Davey Smith G. (1999) *The Widening Gap: Health Inequalities and Policy in Britain*. The Policy Press: Bristol.

Whitley, E., Gunnell, D., Dorling, D. and Davey Smith, G. (1999) Ecological study of social fragmentation, poverty, and suicide. *BMJ*, 319: 1034–7.

WHO (1947) *World Health Organization Constitution*. World Health Organization: Geneva.

Wohl, A.S. (1983) *Endangered Lives: Public Health in Victorian Britain*. Dent: London.

Woods, R. and Shelton, N. (1997) *An Atlas of Victorian Mortality*. Liverpool University Press: Liverpool.

Chapter 3

Mapping and measuring

Chapter summary

We introduce this chapter by considering the characteristics of people which affect health and by asking whether we should study risk at the individual or group level. We discuss the key variables of age, gender and wealth, as well as life course perspectives and clinical measures. We move on to consider the impact of where people live, in terms of 'space and place' and 'time and space'. We then consider data sources: censuses, surveys and routinely recorded data, before asking how these data can be analysed: the recoding of variables, deriving indicators and conducting statistical tests. We end the chapter looking at how these data can be mapped, including chloropleth maps, cartograms and point mapping techniques.

Introduction

In the previous chapter we took a selective, historical view in order to introduce the potential for taking a sociological and geographical perspective on health. Here we begin to look at the range of possibilities for researching social and spatial aspects of health today. This chapter is about the concepts, data and techniques that are frequently used by medical geographers and medical sociologists in their research. The chapter is based around three questions which often need to be addressed as part of a typical piece of research:

1 Who are people? Here we might be interested in their biological, demographic, social and economic characteristics.
2 Where do they live? We might want to know about the material and physical attributes of their location as well as the different associations and meanings attached to different types of place.
3 What has happened to them? We may want to know what has happened to them in terms of their health (such as a heart attack) as well as other events which we may consider to be health-related (such as a bereavement).

At the beginning of the chapter we will explore these three questions by focusing on the conceptual issues they raise and by looking at them from the perspective of medical geography and medical sociology. Following that, we focus on the data sources that are commonly used to answer these questions and a few basic techniques through which these data sources are interrogated and analysed in geographical and sociological research. At the end of the chapter we use two case studies as examples to show how these three questions can be drawn together in answering research questions.

Before we begin it is important to recognize that the questions above form the essence of many other kinds of geography and sociology. It is only a focus on health, particularly with regard to question 3, that makes this chapter about *medical* geography and *medical* sociology. Much of the content of this chapter will thus be applicable and useful for other topics of geographical or sociological study.

It should also be made clear that the research approach outlined in this chapter is solely *quantitative* – that means it is based on the gathering and analysis of numerical information. Qualitative research (based largely on the gathering and analysis of textual and voice-based information) is also extremely valuable in the fields of medical sociology and medical geography. If you want to learn about qualitative research (and it is important that you do understand the breadth and depth of those techniques in order to have a full appreciation of current research) *The Handbook of Qualitative Research* edited by Denzin and Lincoln (1994) is a good place to start (see suggested further reading at the end of this chapter).

This chapter does not provide an exhaustive list of techniques, concepts and methods for geographical and sociological research into health and disease. It does, however, aim to introduce the reader to the more common measures and methods that might be encountered when reading about or beginning to learn, quantitative medical geography and medical sociology.

The reason we ask the three questions above is because the answers to these questions are clearly related to each other and because the connections between the answers to them are the focus of most research questions. These three questions are thus being used with two purposes in mind: first, to help structure the information presented in this chapter; and second, to focus our minds on what medical geographers and medical sociologists actually do when addressing research questions. Try to keep those connections in mind as you read on.

Who are people?

Who are you? It's an intriguing thought... Spend a moment thinking about the aspects of your character, life and personal history that you think might affect your answer and those that might affect your chances of good health and of living for a long time. Perhaps you thought about your age, your sex, how much exercise you take, whether you smoke or not, the kinds of food that you like to eat and whether you have any particular condition or disease? Did you consider other aspects of your life such as where you live, the kind of job you do or might

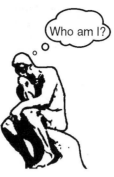

Figure 3.1 Who am I?

do, the kind of job your parents do or did, your genetic inheritance and plain old luck?

Characteristics that affect health

One problem (but also a source of tremendous interest) for researchers concerned with social and spatial aspects of health is that all of the factors mentioned above, amongst many others, legitimately describe 'who people are'. All of them are implicated in an individual's chances of having good or bad health. A key aspect of understanding medical geography and/or medical sociology is selecting and managing the available information about 'who people are'. Which information is most appropriate to answering a particular research question?

It is easier to understand the arguments presented here if you think about them in terms of your own health. Suppose your health were to be 'judged' by someone (in terms of whether it is better or worse than might be expected or than it could be). Which of the characteristics mentioned already do you think should be taken into account when that judgement is made?

Age is a variable (see Box 3.1) that most people would probably consider to be important in considering health. Most people know that your health deteriorates as you get older so that if you have a few aches and pains and are a little bit slower than you used to be, but you are aged 85, that is generally seen as a good state of health for that age. However, aches and pains and slow movement at age 18 are far more likely to be a matter of some medical concern. Do you think that this kind of assumption holds true for other variables that might affect your state of health? Would you make the same kind of judgement for

---

Box 3.1 What is a variable?

A *variable* is any characteristic or attribute which can be measured and can have different values. It 'varies'.

---

people at opposite ends of a scale of wealth, for example? Would somebody, aged 32, with aches and pains, who finds movement increasingly difficult and who is a lawyer, be in a good state of health or poor state of health? What if they were a road sweeper, bricklayer or supermarket shelf-stacker?

Studying risk at the individual or group level

Although the outcomes that we may be studying (such as death) and the data we have may be at the *individual* level, in geographical and sociological research into health we are usually interested in focusing on the *group* level. So rather than looking at individual occupations, we group jobs into categories, such as manual and non-manual occupations. Similarly, we don't compare people in spatial terms using the grid reference of where they live, but in terms of the place in which they live – such as the county or region. We do a similar thing for age – rather than comparing many individuals of different ages (12, 23, 26, 45) we consider age-groups. However, the groups have to make sense for the analysis to make sense. People should be grouped with those most similar to them, so for age, groups such as 0, 1–4… 20–24… and 85+ are common.

An individual's state of health can be influenced by many things (including luck, which is impossible to predict) and individuals can be very different in terms of the way things affect their health. Not all smokers get lung cancer for example, not all athletes live to a great age and not everybody who eats a lot is obese. We are thus more interested in health differences among groups of people, such as those who smoke and those who do not smoke, rather than just one person who smokes and one person who does not.

Medical geography and medical sociology often consider factors in terms of the *risk* they present to health. So for example, while we know that not *all* smokers get lung cancer we know that many *more* smokers get lung cancer than non-smokers (Box 3.2). Smoking *increases the risk* of lung cancer so that a heavy

---

Box 3.2 Four facts about smoking

- The highest recorded level of smoking among men in the UK was 82 per cent in 1948, when surveys were first carried out. Among women, smoking prevalence remained fairly constant between 1948 and 1970 and peaked at 45 per cent in 1966 (Wald, 1991).
- One measure of addiction is how long after waking a person smokes their first cigarette of the day. In 1998, 31 per cent of smokers had their first cigarette within 15 minutes of waking (ONS, 2000).
- A recent US study found that smoking during the teenage years causes permanent genetic changes in the lungs and increases forever the risk of lung cancer, even if the smoker subsequently stops (Wiencke *et al.*, 1999).
- More than one-third of adult Americans have smoked marijuana, with at least 11 million getting high at least once a month (*High Times Magazine*, 1999).

smoker (smoking more than 20 cigarettes a day) is about 30 to 40 times more likely to get lung cancer than a non-smoker.

Working with groups of people who share the same characteristics helps to distinguish differences in their health which are due to chance from those which are the product of actual relationships between the characteristics which they possess and their chances of good or bad health.

To begin to get to grips with this it is useful to think more about variables through which different groups of people can be defined that may best separate those at high risk from those at low risk. At the same time we want our variables to help explain what is most likely to be the underlying influence on those risks. Knowing that people who are very ill are more likely to die soon is not a particularly novel research finding, for instance.

Key variables: age, gender and wealth

Age is a relatively easy variable to understand and is almost always involved in analyses of health. Box 3.3 shows how life expectancy of people of different ages and sexes in England and Wales varied in the mid-1990s. However, age is not as simple a variable as it might at first seem. A person's age indicates how long they have lived, but their date of birth and death also tells us about the historical time that they have lived through. This will give us additional information about the nature of the society in which they lived as well as the events which they might have witnessed. We call the implications of this aspect of age 'cohort' effects.

An example of a cohort effect is the high unemployment experienced by workers during the Great Depression of the 1930s. Another more recent example is the high rate of unemployment experienced by graduating students during the last recession. Students in Britain who graduated during the 1990–93 economic recession, for example, had a very much higher rate of unemployment than those graduating in later years, even though they had the same level of qualification. Spending a significant period of time in unemployment introduces a higher risk of health problems which takes many years to subside. Looking at cohort effects more widely, different generations exposed (or not) to war, very different circumstances of childbirth, different working practices and different types of job all tend to experience different health problems at different rates. Your age is not just about how many birthdays you have celebrated!

Whether people are male or female is almost always involved in analyses of health. This is because differences in health experiences and the risk of death exist between men and women at almost all stages of life, from the cradle to the grave. Generally speaking, men's chances of dying are higher at all points in life but women tend to report higher levels of morbidity (sickness or illness). You might think that whether someone is male or female would be an unambiguous variable, but it is important to understand the ways in which this variable is handled in contemporary research. When we talk about a person's sex we are usually referring to their biological characteristics. When we talk about gender

Box 3.3 Life expectancy by age and sex in England and Wales, 1993–95

This chart shows the number of years a person of each age can expect to live (rounded to whole years). Note how total life expectancy actually increases with age – the longer you live, the longer you are likely to live!

Age	Men	Women
0	74	79
1	74	79
2	73	78
3	72	77
4	71	76
5–9	70	75
10–14	65	70
15–19	60	65
20–24	55	60
25–29	40	55
30–34	45	50
35–39	41	45
40–44	36	40
45–49	31	36
50–54	27	32
55–59	22	27
60–64	18	22
65–69	15	18
70–74	11	15
75–79	9	11
80–84	7	9
85+	5	6

Note: rounded to whole years.

Source: ONS (1997). © Crown Copyright 2000.

on the other hand, we are referring not only to biological differences but also to the social and cultural aspects of being male or female (see Box 3.4). Throughout life we are socialized into what is considered to be acceptable and appropriate behaviour for our sex – we are engendered. In western societies, for example, girls are expected to hold the feminine traits of passivity, sensitivity and caring for others, whereas boys are expected to have masculine traits of independence, being active and being emotionally hardy. What is considered appropriate masculine and feminine traits will vary from place to place, and over time.

Some have argued that gender is a 'false dichotomy' and recently this simple dichotomy has been problematized and explored in much greater depth. A growing body of research looks at gender as a far more complex 'spectrum'

Box 3.4 Let's talk about sex

Sex is usually taken to refer to the *biological* division between female and male.

Gender is used to refer to the learnt social and cultural aspects of the difference between feminine and masculine. The emphasis here is upon the socially constructed aspects of femininity and masculinity.

---

rather than just a straightforward biological division. Indices that can describe the strength of a person's masculinity and femininity have allowed gender to be described in more complex terms. Interestingly, different scores on these indices appear to be strongly related to the chances of good health, or to health-related behaviour, independently of 'biological' gender.

Despite understanding that gender is complex, for practical reasons, in the majority of quantitative analyses of health, we usually use a simple dichotomous variable referring to whether someone is male or female. While we do this, however, we should bear in mind that gender is about very much more than biology.

Beyond age and sex there is a whole host of variables that describe characteristics of people's lives and that are related to health. How well-off people are in socio-economic terms is a crucial variable because in every society, people are differentiated by the wealth that they possess or have access to. In western societies people's socio-economic resources are a key feature determining the nature and quality of their lives. This is also important in that medical sociologists and medical geographers consistently find strong relationships between socio-economic indicators and health; debate abounds as to precisely why and how wealth and poverty influence the likelihood of good health or the chances of premature death. Section II of this book addresses that debate.

It is important to grasp the various dimensions by which someone can be better or worse off as this tells us a lot about the conditions of their life (see Box 3.5). This issue is also related to how we collect and analyse data. It should be clear that we are not only referring to the amount of money that someone may have, but more widely to the pool of resources which they own or to which they have access.

When we talk about people in society being better or worse off we also invoke notions of other less tangible assets, such as education, the resources (financial or otherwise) that may be offered by friends or colleagues, the security and stability furnished by property ownership or from having a regular job and a whole host of other 'assets'. There is a dispute in the research literature about whether it is the *material* or the *social* aspects of wealth that are most directly related to health. This is difficult to unravel because the one usually accompanies the other. However, what seems most likely is that different aspects of wealth make different contributions to the health or health-related behaviour that is experienced by an individual.

One final point to remember at this stage is that how well-off or poor an individual is according to these different dimensions is likely to change through

Box 3.5 Rich or poor? Measuring socio-economic resources

1 **Income** refers to the *flow* of money an individual (or household) receives weekly, monthly or annually. For many people their main source of income is through paid work; others receive income from benefit payments or from pensions and other investments. Levels of income can fluctuate over the long or short term. Income is not measured in the UK census, but is captured by the US census. Many people are reticent about divulging their income and so income data are often relatively unreliable.

2 **Wealth** refers to the *stock* of money that a person has (such as money in a bank account or invested in stocks and shares) as well as the value of the assets that they own. Much of all wealth in Britain is held in the form of housing wealth – if a person owns or has partly paid off a mortgage on their own home, how much it is worth is an indicator of wealth. It is very difficult to collect reliable information on wealth.

3 **Social class or socio-economic group** another way in which we can learn about a person's socio-economic position is to find out about their employment status (whether they work or not) and if they do work, what kind of occupation they have. Occupations can then be divided into **occupational social classes** or into **socio-economic groups**. These occupationally based classes correlate closely with both income and wealth – those in higher social classes tend to have higher incomes and hold more wealth than those further down the social scale. It is much easier to collect information on occupation than on income and wealth. (In Chapter 4 we examine social class in Britain, and its relationship to health, in more detail.)

4 **Amenity access** an alternative measure of socio-economic resources can be constructed from looking at the amenities to which people have access. Common examples of amenities are: cars, central heating systems and having toilets inside the property. This form of measurement is good for identifying people at the bottom of the socio-economic scale.

5 **Geographical location** equates residential location with wealth through the assumption that richer folk live in richer neighbourhoods. This can be useful when data are not available at the individual level but are available at the neighbourhood or area level.

time. Income, for example, is closely related to age; the attainment of professional qualifications that tend to put an individual at the top of the income scale, takes time. People tend to accumulate wealth over their lifetime, for example, as they pay their mortgage to buy their own home or save money from their income. Conversely, people can become relatively poor quite quickly, because of adverse events such as redundancy or separation.

Life course perspectives

Much of the data collected for or used in health-related research is *cross-sectional* – it has been collected at one point in time and is thus a kind of 'snapshot' of one particular time and place. However, these data do not allow us to look at changes over time, such as whether an individual becomes poorer or wealthier and how that affects their health. Nor do they allow us to look at the effects of the *accumulation* of socio-economic advantage or disadvantage on health. In recent years a body of research has emerged which shows that there is a link between early life socio-economic circumstances, in childhood and even at the foetal stage, and health outcomes experienced later in life. (See Kuh and Beh-Shlomo, 1997, for an excellent overview of current evidence and debates.) If we are trying to understand relationships between the characteristics of a group and their health at one particular point in time, we should also endeavour to understand the nature of the life and experiences which that group has had prior to the point at which we are studying them. If they are unemployed now, have they always been unemployed? They may be relatively well-to-do now, but what were their childhood socio-economic circumstances? However, we often do not have as much information about a person's lifetime circumstances as we would like.

A stark contrast between childhood and adult life circumstances provides an unusual but interesting example of this difficulty in health research. Elvis Presley grew up in conditions of extreme relative poverty but at the time of his death he was one of the richest men in the world. Some have argued that it was the imprint of deprived childhood circumstances which was ultimately responsible for the characteristics of his untimely demise at the age of 42. If Elvis had been rich all his life, that life may well have been considerably longer, but considerably less remarkable (personal communication, George Davey Smith).

Deciding how to deal with the mismatch between available data and the nature of a research question is a key aspect of being a good medical geographer or medical sociologist. Often there is no easy solution. The researcher can only state the limitations of the data available to them and be clear about how these may have affected their results. The results of any study, however, should be put into the context of the findings of other research on that topic – how do they compare? Each study can be seen as a part of a much larger puzzle.

More variables of interest

There are literally hundreds of characteristics which an individual might have and which are related to their chances of experiencing good health, but of course we do not have the space to review them all here. The variables chosen for inclusion in a study will derive from the specific research question being posed, the findings of previous studies, and the availability of data. Two important and common variables which we have only briefly referred to as yet, but which you will no doubt encounter when reading medical geography or medical sociology, are unemployment and smoking. There is a large volume of literature that explores the relationship between unemployment and health (see Box 3.6 for some details).

Smoking is the characteristic that almost everyone now knows is related to bad health. There is no doubt about it, smoking is bad for you (see Box 3.7 for more details). Like other characteristics we have looked at, recording the

---

Box 3.6 Four facts about unemployment and health

- Many studies have found that unemployed people have worse health than those in work. There has been a vigorous debate about this – is it unemployment that causes ill health or are ill people just more likely to become unemployed? In fact, the evidence now suggests that although ill people *are* more likely to become unemployed, unemployment *is* bad for your health.
- The first convincing evidence of a causal relationship between unemployment and ill-health came from an analysis of a British longitudinal study in the mid-1980s (Moser *et al.*, 1987).
- Several studies have found higher rates of smoking and alcohol use and poorer diet among unemployed people but a study of British men aged 40–59 years found no evidence that they increased their smoking or drinking on becoming unemployed, though they were more likely to gain weight. The men who became unemployed had higher levels of smoking and alcohol consumption to begin with (Power and Estaugh, 1990; Lee *et al.*, 1991; Morris *et al.*, 1992; Bartley, 1994).
- In Australia, children whose parents were unemployed were reported to have around 26 per cent more serious chronic illnesses than those with one or more of their parents in employment (Mathers, 1995).

---

smoking status of someone is rather more difficult than it first appears. How would you describe your 'smoking status'? Have you ever smoked? (*Really?*) Perhaps you are a 'non-smoker' – but the chances are that you may have smoked at least one or two cigarettes in your life, and what about passive smoking? Do you live or work in an environment in which you are exposed to 'second-hand' smoke? What if you used to be a smoker but then gave up? Do you believe that the effects of this habit are still with you and affecting your health? A view across the life course makes things even more complicated.

Box 3.7 Four more facts about smoking and disease

- It has been estimated that, on average, one cigarette knocks about 11 minutes off your life (Shaw *et al.*, 2000).
- Smoking causes around 82 per cent of all deaths from lung cancer, around 83 per cent of all deaths from bronchitis and emphysema and around 25 per cent of all deaths from heart disease in America (ASH, 2000).
- Less than 10 per cent of lung cancer patients survive five years after diagnosis (ASH, 2000).
- Women who smoke and take the contraceptive pill have 10 times the risk of a heart attack, stroke or other cardiovascular disease compared with those who take the pill but are non-smokers. Smoking has also been linked with an increased likelihood of menstrual problems (ASH, 2000).

Clinical characteristics

Another way in which medical geography and medical sociology describe 'who people are' is the use of biological or clinical information. Clinical data refer to measurements of physiology and biology and may include characteristics such as height, weight, blood pressure (see Box 3.8), respiratory function (how easily you can breathe) and, increasingly, attributes of blood or even of genetic material. It would be wrong to assume that all (or even most) medical geography or medical sociology makes use of these clinical measures, but their use does perhaps provide an interesting feature which distinguishes much medical sociology and medical geography from their wider disciplines.

The relationship between these clinical data, which describe the physical status of the body, and the characteristics described above (such as smoking status or social class) is fascinating. In some ways the variables that describe characteristics about the way in which people live their lives (whether they smoke or not, what their job is, etc.) describe the context for the world in which the 'body' exists. The concoctions of fluids and cells which we all comprise and which are described by 'clinical' data, exist in different physical and social environments which are themselves described by other characteristics.

It is important to be aware of the very different nature of data drawn from self-reported information about people's personal characteristics and their health status and clinical data that need to be collected by qualified medical staff; these types of measurement are far more 'invasive'. Although this might seem to be one of the more 'scientific' aspects of health research, we need to be

---

Box 3.8 What does blood pressure mean?

- Each time a nurse or doctor 'takes' your blood pressure, they are recording two measurements: your systolic pressure and your diastolic pressure. If the two measurements were 110 and 70, they would be written as '110/70'.
- Your systolic pressure (the first and higher number) is the pressure or force the heart places on the walls of your blood vessels as it is pumping with each heartbeat.
- Diastolic pressure (the second and lower number) is the lowest pressure the blood places on the walls of your blood vessels when the heart is relaxed between beats.
- Both of these measurements are important. A high systolic pressure indicates strain on the blood vessels when the heart is attempting to pump blood into your bloodstream. If your diastolic pressure is high, it means that your blood vessels have little chance to relax between heartbeats.
- Occasional high blood pressure is common. Exercise, anxiety or nervousness can cause a high reading (seeing a nurse or physician for the first time can cause this response). Untreated sustained high blood pressure can increase your risk of premature strokes and heart attacks.
- Blood pressure is said to be 'high' when your reading is continuously more than about 140/90.

aware of the ideological context in which such measurement is conducted. People living in western society are increasingly aware, and wary, of developments in the fields of genetic technology and the desire of companies (notably insurance groups) to gain access to genetic information about individuals. This adds a potential new realm of concern to the collection of clinical information. Traditionally, people in western societies dislike giving information about their financial circumstances; they may become increasingly reluctant to give anyone the opportunity to assess their genetic circumstances. Remember, research takes place in the context of a wider society and that means we need to be acutely aware of the ways in which people will react to our requests for the information we need in order to understand their health circumstances.

Section summary

This section has introduced two key ideas. First, there is a whole host of variables that might be used to describe 'who people are' in this context. These include aspects of their behaviour, their socio-economic status and their biology. Second, the measurement of these variables is not always as straightforward as it might first appear. There is a tension between keeping the information collected simple (and in a form that can be analysed) and ensuring that it captures the true nature and variety of people's characteristics. In addition, the dimension of time cannot be ignored in health research and if we really want to understand the ways in which the nature of people's lives are related to their health, it is vital to understand how that relationship has changed (or remained the same) through time. Quantitative medical geographers and medical sociologists rely on data to fuel their analyses. Their results are determined by the data available to them and the ways in which they choose to analyse those data. The best social science takes place where there is an understanding of the relationship between the nature of the questions being asked, the mechanisms that might be at play, and the data available to help answer them.

Where do people live?

Why would medical geographers and medical sociologists want to know where people live? The key reasons are to investigate whether there are geographical patterns of ill-health, and if there are, to explore the relationship between area of residence (or work, or school, etc.) and the chances of good or bad health.

Knowing where people live allows us to monitor the health of particular populations defined by their collective residence or congregation in the same area. Differences in the health of populations who live in different places are taken very seriously, not least because they relate to issues of equity in health care and in health outcomes. These between-area differences in health can operate at a number of levels. For example, if the people who live close to a chemical plant appear to have a higher risk of developing an unpleasant disease than do people who live a long way away from it, there are profound implications for the plant, the population and government who has responsibility for public safety. There are a myriad of examples where close proximity to a source of pollution has been associated with an unusual level of ill-health amongst a population (see reference to the film *Erin Brockovich* at the end of the chapter).

Between-area differences in health which are not directly due to a specific source of pollution or another identifiable environmental factor are also important to research because they may reveal systematic differences in the life chances of different kinds of people. In Britain, for example, there is a great deal of debate about the 'north–south divide', with the north typically represented as a less affluent and 'sicker' part of the country (see Chapter 4 for a more detailed discussion). In New York, for example, some parts of the city are very clearly less affluent and 'sicker' than others – the Bronx is one example. These different types of between-area health differences are important in that they imply different responses for their alleviation. A chemical plant can be closed down, but the nature of society is much harder to change. Many politicians in western society espouse the principle of equal opportunity for all members of society. It is a serious issue if life in one part of a country appears to hold a much higher risk of disease or shortened life span. The relationship between residential location and health is thus an important, and sometimes highly political, one. Medical geographers are equipped with a wide range of techniques to detect and explore between-area differences in health.

A second reason for being interested in 'where people live' is that such information can be useful to derive information about them that we cannot obtain from other sources. There is an old adage that is particularly pertinent in geography: 'birds of a feather flock together'. This saying suggests that similar types of people tend to live in similar places. Often this is not so much a matter of individual choice, but because they could not afford to live elsewhere (would you live where you do now if you had significantly more money?). There is an entire industry dedicated to assigning characteristics to people based on the kind of neighbourhood in which they live (this is called 'geodemographics'). In Box 3.5 we saw how an indicator of income can be assigned to people based on the neighbourhood in which they live. In medical geography we make many other such assumptions based on our knowledge about where people live.

Where do you live?

Where do you live? The majority of us have a single place which we call home. That fixed point can be referenced, perhaps most obviously by a postal address, but also by a map reference or some other kind of precise physical measurement. One common way by which we communicate 'where we live' in our day-to-day lives is by giving people our postcode (see Box 3.9), or zipcode. Before we consider the ways in which 'where people live' can be described or measured we should think a little bit more about the nature of this kind of information (see Figure 3.2).

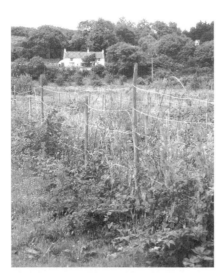
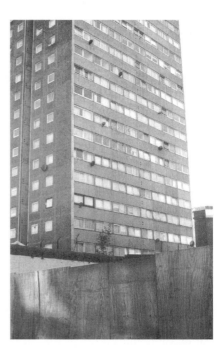

Figure 3.2 Where do you live?

Source: Photographs by Mary Shaw.

We can think about where people live in two ways. First there is a physical point in space which describes a person's residential location. This is the place which we call 'home', where most of our worldly possessions are kept, and where we usually return to sleep, eat and rest. Second, there is the area within which that home-point exists. The boundaries of that physical area may be set in a number of ways but most often we refer to a neighbourhood, a district, a city, a county or state, or even a country. Medical geographers and medical

---

Box 3.9 The UK postcode (e.g. OX7 2AT)

- The UK postcode system is hierarchical, consisting of postcode *areas*, postcode *districts* and postcode *sectors* which together make up a *unit* postcode.
- The *area* code consists of one or two letters, representing the main town or city of the area – for example 'OX' (Oxford) covers most of Oxfordshire.
- The *district* code is designated by adding a number from 0 to 99 to the area code – for example 'OX7'.
- The district code is followed by a space and then the postcode *sector* which is a single digit from 0 to 9 (e.g. OX7 2). There are around 9,000 postcode sectors in the UK, each containing about 2,000 households.
- The unit postcode is completed by the addition of two letters. This identifies approximately 15–30 households or one building if it receives on average more than 25 items of mail per day.

---

sociologists often use these boundaries as a means of grouping people together with the implication that shared residence within those boundaries has some kind of meaning. This is a very common assumption in the whole of western society (the term 'western' is of course geographical itself). Think how often you have heard a stereotypical analysis of 'a New Yorker', 'a Londoner' or 'a Northerner'. Society often makes judgements (or forms stereotypes) about people, grouping them together according to their area of residence. Medical geography and medical sociology do the same kind of thing, although they sometimes use a little more information to do it.

Space and place

Geographers are particularly keen to make the distinction between the definition of area that is primarily spatial (i.e. based on some kind of administrative or physical boundary and called *space*) and one that is social (i.e. takes account of the meaning of that particular area for a particular individual, or group of people and is called *place*). A good way to understand this distinction is to think about your own home. The place you come from has particular meaning for you. It has a character built up from your experiences of living there, your knowledge of the area and, importantly, your knowledge of and interaction with your co-residents who may be family, friends, acquaintances or strangers. This is what the quote in Box 3.10 is aiming to address. The crucial distinction between place and space is that it is possible for two people to come from or live in the same physical space but for them to experience it, think about it and live there in completely different ways – to come from different *places*. Sharing physical space (area) is not the same as sharing social space (place). This also has profound implications for a researcher trying to study an area that they may have never visited and about which they know little. The description of that area from available data might lead to a particular impression of that area, but this impression may be very different from that which the residents themselves have. Qualitative research methods are particularly suited to teasing out the meanings which people ascribe to places.

Time and space

In the same way that time is an important aspect to consider when collecting data about 'who people are', time is important when considering 'where you

Box 3.10 A word about space and place

We are located in 'space', but we act in 'place'. Furthermore, 'places' are spaces that are valued. The distinction is rather like that between a 'house' and a 'home'; a house might keep out the wind and the rain, but a home is where we live.

(Harrison and Dourish, 1996)

live'. Migration (the movement of people from one place to another) has profound consequences for medical geography and medical sociology (half of Chapter 6 in this book is dedicated to the subject). Think about the examples we have used in this section. When trying to determine whether a chemical factory is the source of pollution it would be vital to know whether the people who became ill had lived near the factory for a reasonable amount of time, whether they had come there from somewhere else (which might have been the true source of their illness) or whether other people who used to live nearby but who moved away also became ill.

'Selective migration' is the term given to the process through which an area's population may be healthier or sicker than average because people who are healthier or sicker than the average have either moved in or moved out. Suppose for example that there is an economic collapse in a particular district and employment prospects there are bleak. Those who are able to move out may well do so, leaving behind those less able to move (perhaps including the infirm). Research might identify that area as having a higher number of ill people than average but in this case that may have little to do with the nature of the area itself: the situation has been created by the selective movement of different types of people. The history of 'where you live' is an important aspect of medical geography and medical sociology.

However, just as it is important to make a distinction between space and place it is important to make the distinction between time and history. People can live at the same time but have very different personal histories. Time and space are the metrics we use to locate people and pinpoint the moments in which they have lived or moved. Place and history describe how people view their location, movement and passage through time. Being able to take account of your own prejudices and perceptions when thinking about time and space, histories and place, is a vital part of being a good researcher.

Section summary

There are many different ways to describe where people live but the most commonly employed method in medical geography is to make reference to an *areal unit* within which the individual resides. That areal unit is usually defined by some set or sets of administrative unit(s). Assumptions are often made that people who live within the same administrative unit share characteristics or are at least exposed to similar influences on their health. Changes in residential location are important. Place is different from space. Time is not history.

What has happened to people?

Medical geographers and medical sociologists are primarily interested in health and health-related outcomes, including behaviour (such as smoking, healthy eating or unprotected sex). 'Outcome' is the word we use to describe the vari-

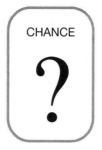

Figure 3.3 Chance.

able that we are interested in studying and understanding, whether that be someone's state of health (including whether they are alive or dead) or elements of their health-related behaviour.

We can divide information about what has happened to people into biological and social categories in the same way that we divided information about 'who people are'. Again, there is an enormous range of life events and health outcomes that might be explored under these headings. Rather than investigate all of these we will take a brief look at different types of outcomes and use these examples to lead into an exploration of data sources and analysis techniques which will form the rest of the chapter.

Death

The final health outcome is death. Data about the timing, location and nature of death and the deceased form a very common element of medical geography and medical sociology. The number of deaths that occur among a population, expressed in relation to its size and composition, is a very common way of assessing that population's health. This measure is called the *mortality rate*. Information about the cause of death is also often analysed, and the mortality rate for specific causes can also be calculated. Often the risk of death from a specific cause is related to individual characteristics (see Figure 3.3) but social and spatial patterns are also apparent. Medical geographers and medical sociologists often referred to death as 'mortality'. We will look in more detail at how mortality data are collected and analysed later in the chapter (see Box 3.11).

Box 3.11 Mortality rate, or death rate

Number of deaths in a population or group divided by the number of people in that population or group.

Death rates are usually calculated for specific age-groups, for each sex, and can be calculated for specific causes of death.

Illness

Medical geographers and medical sociologists are also interested in illness, which is often referred to as 'morbidity'. Morbidity can be measured in a variety of ways. *Clinical measures* are those collected by a health professional. This can include information on diagnoses made by a doctor, such as a cancer diagnosis, as well as measurements, such as blood pressure (see Box 3.8). Information on illness can also be *self-reported*, that is, an individual respondent, typically in a survey or interview, gives an assessment of their own health. Data on clinical measures often give far more detail about the state of people's health – in terms of the biomedical model they are more 'scientific' – but they are generally far more time-consuming and expensive to collect than self-reported measures.

Because of issues related to the practicalities of collecting data, self-reported measures of morbidity in medical geography and medical sociology are commonplace, but often problematic and sometimes controversial. Some people may consider that they are 'healthy' but a medical investigation might label them as 'diseased'. For example, many people who have what is considered to be 'high' blood pressure are unaware of this. Similarly, if you ask somebody whether they have a particular disease you may well get a different answer from that which a doctor would give if he or she were asked to assess their state of health. Good examples of diseases for which a doctor's diagnosis and an individual's self-reporting might vary are: heart problems, asthma and depression. Who really knows more about a person's state of health: a doctor or the individual concerned? How reliable is an individual's own perception of their state of health? How reliable is the doctor's?

In addition to specific illness information, medical geographers and medical sociologists are often interested in more general measures of health. A very common question used to capture the general state of health prompts survey respondents to reveal whether they think that their health is poor, average, good or very good. What kind of things do you think would influence your response? Do you have a cold, any minor injury, a long-term illness, or are you just feeling particularly happy or particularly sad? One problem with this type of health information is that the response an individual gives is prone to all sorts of influences. Some people are naturally more pessimistic than others, while others would deny that there is anything wrong with them at all, even when medical science would suggest that there is little hope for them! Sociologists have a special term for a pessimistic attitude, 'negative affectivity', and the development of techniques to try to adjust statistical analyses for negative affectivity is an evolving field within this discipline. However, despite these problems with measures of self-reported health, such measures tend to correlate highly with other health outcomes, such as the use of health services or mortality.

Box 3.12 describes a commonly used self-reported health measure, the General Health Questionnaire (GHQ). The GHQ relates to mental health, rather than physical health.

Box 3.12 The General Health Questionnaire (GHQ)

- The GHQ measures how a respondent feels their *present* state of mind (i.e. over the past two weeks) compares with their *usual* state. It aims to distinguish circumstances: inability to carry out one's normal 'healthy' functions and the appearance of new phenomena of a distressing nature.
- It is a self-administered test aimed at detecting psychiatric disorders in a community setting. It was designed to be easy to administer, fairly short and acceptable to respondents.
- There are various versions available with different numbers of questions, the GHQ-60, GHQ-28, GHQ-30 and GHQ-12.

Possible responses are: Better than usual; Same as usual; Worse than usual; Much worse than usual.

The actual questions of the GHQ are subject to copyright restrictions. For more information contact the company which owns the questions, NFER-NELSON (http://www.nfer-nelson. co.uk/) or see Goldberg and Williams (1988).

Some researchers prefer to use self-reported data to describe health because they are more interested in how people feel than in how medical science would categorize them. In trying to understand behaviour and how people experience their lives it can be more important to capture feelings or perceptions than to make a clinical diagnosis. Others prefer to deal in clinical and biological measures of health such as blood pressure, lung performance, height and weight. There are many issues to consider when opting for self-reported or clinical measures, but the nature of the research question being asked will be a key determinant. In the practical world of research, issues such as cost (employing skilled staff to measure or diagnose the health of large survey populations is extremely expensive), time, the pre-existence of readily available data and willingness of a survey population to be clinically examined all contribute to the choice of health outcome being studied.

Other life events

In addition to information about the health of a population or individual, 'what has happened to people' can include significant life events such as giving birth, getting married or divorced, or being made redundant. Events such as these can have an impact on health in both the short and long term. A huge range of information can be gathered to describe the circumstances and details of these kinds of life event. An example of a study that considered life events that might be stressful is shown in Box 3.13.

Section summary

It may be becoming apparent that our three-question division is somewhat artificial, and it is. To understand the health that people enjoy, the ill-health from

---

Box 3.13 Stressful life events and self-rated health

In a study set in East and West Berlin shortly after reunification in 1991, Hillen *et al.* (2000) investigated the effects on self-reported health of living under different political systems. They found evidence that people who had lived in East Berlin had poorer self-rated health, and that this was related to stressful life events. These were the stressful life events that were measured, as they were thought to be most pertinent to that population at that particular time:

- Caregiver to a dependent person during the past year.
- Worries about family members.
- Death of a spouse within the past year.
- Divorce within the past year.
- Change of residence within the past year.
- Insufficient recognition at the workplace.
- Current unemployment.
- Threatening loss of employment.
- Dissatisfaction with financial situation.
- Feelings of being overcharged for goods and services.

---

which they suffer and the circumstances of their death is a tremendous task. A full understanding is only possible when the health outcome is placed in the context of the life lived, and that includes a person's history, the circumstances of their birth and of their development in childhood and through adult life. However, the limitations of the research process require medical geographers and medical sociologists to make choices. It is simply not possible to capture all the data that would adequately describe the vast complexity of a person's journey through life. So far in this chapter we have outlined the types of data that are commonly employed in research of this kind but it is as important to bear in mind those data that are left out of analyses as it is to understand those that are included.

In the next section we review a number of commonly employed data sets, and then look at how these are combined in some analyses commonly conducted by medical geographers and medical sociologists.

Data sources: censuses, surveys and routinely recorded data

It is well beyond the scope of this chapter, or even a whole book, to document every single data source that medical geographers or medical sociologists might wish to access (see Kerrison and Macfarlane, 2000). Instead we are going to look at three broad types of data set. Remember, research of this kind needs information not only specifically about the health of the population but also about the context for that health, i.e. the broader nature of society. The three broad types of data we cover here are: censuses, surveys and routinely recorded data sets.

Censuses

Censuses are unique because they are the only instance when data are collected, in theory at least, from a complete population, rather than from a sample of that population. In the United Kingdom and the United States population censuses are carried out every ten years and form the basis for a great many social and economic policy decisions by both central and local government.

The census is conducted and controlled by the state and this has both advantages and disadvantages. The advantages are that censuses are, on the whole, well funded, and thus have a social and spatial coverage not matched by any other survey. As completing a census form is a legal requirement, they also tend to have very high response rates and thus lead to very accurate data. The disadvantages stem from the scale of the process (it is almost impossible to collect information from *everybody* in a census) and from the necessary limitations on the range and nature of questions that can be asked. Although we know that even the best census 'misses' some people, a census is still the closest thing we have to a common set of questions to which everyone (or most people) in the country has responded (see www.census.ac.uk and www.census.gov).

Censuses are a vital source of information for medical geographers and medical sociologists for two reasons: (a) they provide basic information about the composition of the population and their location (for example, counts of people by age and sex in each area), and (b) they provide some information about the health of everyone in the country. The British and US census systems currently differ in the information which they gather about health. In addition, the questions tend to change from census to census, although they are almost always of a very general nature. The information about the size and nature of the population in different areas that can be derived from censuses is extremely valuable for medical geographers. In any study of the health differences between different parts of a country, variations between the basic characteristics of those populations need to be taken into account (see Chapter 5 for more details). A census provides a readily accessible, reliable and standard source of that information.

Surveys

Most medical geographers or medical sociologists are very likely to use survey data of some kind in the course of their work. (Box 3.14 helps to distinguish between censuses and surveys.) Surveys come in many different forms and sizes and thus the term 'survey' is a very general label. A defining aspect of survey data, however, is that they are constructed through the use of a sample. Because it is usually too time-consuming and expensive to collect data on a whole population, survey researchers collect information from a sample of that population. A census is a special kind of survey where everyone in the population is surveyed, and in that case the population and the sample are (almost) the same thing. Sample surveys are used not only because they involve less effort, but because if the sample is representative of the population, then it is not necessary to collect information from the total population. If the sample is of sufficient

---

Box 3.14 What is a survey and how does it relate to a census?

- The term **survey** describes a means of gathering information from a *sample* of individuals where the *sample* is a fraction or subgroup of the wider population being studied. For example, a *sample* of voters is questioned in advance of an election to determine how the public perceives the candidates and the issues, and how they might cast their vote. In a **census**, the aim is to gather information from *everyone* in the population, not just a sample.
- The size of a sample depends on the purpose of the survey.
- Surveys can be conducted in lots of different ways: over the telephone, by mail, by e-mail or in person.
- A representative sample means that the results can be reliably extrapolated from the sample to the wider population.
- A sample should not be selected haphazardly – including only those persons who are most convenient to the researcher or who volunteer to participate in the research. The sample can be designed so that each person in the population will have an equal chance of being included in the sample. It is this characteristic that ensures that a sample is actually representative. This is referred to as **random sampling**. Remember, random sampling is not haphazard, but is highly structured and controlled.
- To refer to the size of a sample we use the notation n. For example, $n = 1,543$.

---

size, and representative of the population, then the information obtained from the sample can be generalized to the population as a whole (Box 3.15).

For example, suppose we are interested in the health behaviours of students in the United States. We have two possible approaches to gathering this information – we could ask every student in the United States to fill in our survey questionnaire, or we could ask a much smaller group of students our set of questions, and use the answers they give as an indication of the variety of responses which all students in the United States might make. The obvious issue here is how well our subgroup of students will capture the variety of responses that the whole US student population might make. This issue of how *representative* a sample is of its population is thus a crucial aspect of the survey method. If a sample is not representative of the population that we are trying to describe then the results tell us only about that sample, and cannot be used more generally (unless they are weighted). When interpreting the results of any survey research, always look for evidence of the representativeness of the sample.

Box 3.15 Population and Sample

Population refers to the total of individuals or units under investigation, from which a sample is drawn.

Sample A subset of the population about which a researcher collects information.

Earlier in the chapter we discussed the fact that health behaviours and health outcomes can vary according to certain characteristics of the population, such as age and gender. Health behaviours and health outcomes can also vary across different locations. If our survey is concerned with measuring variation in health behaviours or health outcomes along those lines then it is vital to capture an appropriate representation of the population in terms of its characteristics and spatial dispersion. For example, it would be useless to try to find out how health varies among the student population across the whole of the United States by asking questions in only one or two colleges. Likewise, we would not obtain a representative sample if we ignored, for example, richer students, black students or male students, as we know that those are likely to be important characteristics in relation to health outcome. If a survey is aiming to say something about the health of a specific population, the people who actually answer the questions must constitute a 'mini' version of that specific population.

Primary and secondary survey data

It is important to distinguish between *primary* and *secondary* survey data. Primary data are those that are constructed by (or for) a specific piece of research which is being undertaken by the researcher in question. Secondary data are those that are not constructed with a specific research purpose in mind, or by the research team in question. Suppose for example that we are interested in understanding the sexual health of young people. Primary survey data might be information we collect, perhaps in schools or in the homes of young people, by asking specific questions which relate precisely to our research questions. We might also use secondary data, which may be derived from surveys that have already been undertaken (by other researchers) and that included questions of relevance to this research. Secondary data can be gathered from publications, data archives or directly from the primary researcher. Many primary data sets are thus reused as secondary data by other research teams. There is a tradition of depositing primary data collected as part of specific research projects into *data archives* to which the wider academic world has access. The effect of the growing amount of archived data, much of which is available or catalogued online, is to greatly increase the range of data sets available to researchers. As our capacity and willingness to analyse large volumes of data from a variety of sources increases, the utility of having common sets of questions through which data sets may be linked together becomes more obvious. We will return to this point again shortly. Before that let us consider further subdivisions of survey data.

Types of survey

Following from the distinction between primary and secondary data is the nature of the questions that the survey poses. Often large-scale secondary data sets cover a wide range of health-related questions, perhaps asking information about the social and economic characteristics of the survey respondents, but they tend to have breadth rather than depth. Many primary data sets, on the other hand, cover a more specific topic, being focused on one particular disease or health behaviour in much greater detail. This distinction between general and more specific data is often mirrored in the geography of such surveys. Some very detailed surveys are set in a specific geographical location (such as a particular town or city) and therefore offer a good picture of particular health problems in that area. Other larger-scale surveys may aim to cover a much greater geographical area, such as a region or a whole country, and thus there are fewer respondents in any particular area but their geographical spread is much greater.

Another aspect of surveys to consider is the way in which they deal with or include time. The vast majority of surveys are what is called *cross-sectional*, that is, they take place at one point in time and provide a 'snapshot' of people's lives and their health-related behaviour or outcome at that single point in time. However, many aspects of health have developed over a long period of time, as we have already noted in some detail. Imagine asking about employment status in a survey questionnaire. If a woman says that she is unemployed, can we tell whether she has never worked or was made redundant one day or ten years before the survey date?

There are two ways to capture time in survey data. First, you could repeatedly visit the same set of individuals throughout their lives. These kind of surveys are called *longitudinal* or *cohort* studies. By repeatedly surveying members of the study sample, sometimes referred to as a *panel*, the ways in which their lives and health develop can be captured and monitored. Although this is probably the most accurate way of watching someone's life unfold and is often used for deriving conclusions about the relationships between life events, individual characteristics and health outcomes, it is also one of the most expensive and difficult types of survey to conduct. A commitment to this kind of research requires very long-term funding, the ability to keep in touch with or trace the survey respondents throughout their lives and also the ability to analyse the very much more complex data that stem from this kind of survey process.

The second means of capturing time is to ask retrospective questions in the survey questionnaire. To continue our example, we would ask how long the woman had been unemployed. Although this may sound very much easier than trying to follow someone through time and repeatedly surveying them, the accuracy of the data collected using this method is often called into question because we are relying on people's memories. People may not accurately remember details such as in which year they had an accident or got a job, or what their birth weight was (if indeed they ever knew). One development that improves our ability to collect retrospective data is the *life grid* method of interviewing. Life grids construct a time-line for the respondent (an interviewee) using key dates such as the birth of a child, the death of a political figure or the beginning or end of a war. These are used as markers to aid the construction of a more accurate chronology of personal life events. So for example, if someone was being asked about their work history, and the interviewer was trying to establish the amount of time spent working in a particular occupation, reference might be made to a point in time specified on the life grid: 'were you still working at that factory when your third child was born?'

Despite the growing acceptance that the development of someone's life is of profound importance in determining their risks of illness or death, the vast majority of survey data are cross-sectional and contain limited information about how the survey respondent's life developed through time; some still ignore the dimension of time completely.

Health survey data, then, are drawn from a sample of the population (i.e. not everyone in that population responds to the questionnaire or the interview) and may cover health in either general or specific terms. They differ from a census, which asks everybody in the population the same set of general questions and which is not specifically dedicated to capturing information about health.

Routinely recorded data

The third and final source of data we consider here is that of *routinely recorded data*. Routinely recorded sources usually stem from contact with the state or with medical services and in that sense differ markedly from survey data in which contact with respondents is initiated by the researcher. The most obvious example of a routinely recorded data source is mortality records, which derive from information given on death certificates (see Figure 3.4).

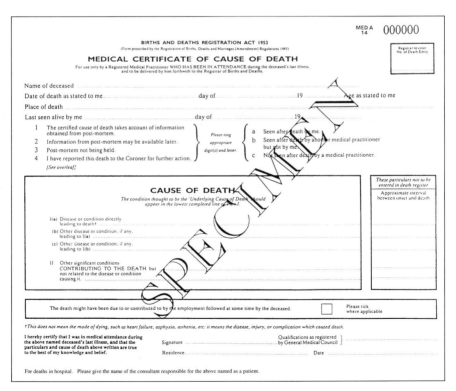

Figure 3.4 England and Wales Death Certificate, 1998.

Source: Mortality Statistics. Series DH1 No. 29 National Statistics © Crown copyright.

Box 3.16 What is the ICD?

The International Classification of Diseases is a global standard system used to classify mortality information for statistical purposes. Most medical geographers or medical sociologists encounter the ICD in mortality data. The ICD is used as a standard means of indicating cause of death. In the table below, an example of ICD codes and their meaning is provided. ICD codes are periodically updated (the ones below are from the ninth revision).

Top five leading causes of death – Utah County Health Department

Cause of death	ICD–9 Codes	1986–88 Rate	1989–91 Rate	1992–94 Rate
1 Diseases of heart	(390–398; 402; 404–429)	86.4 (701)	78.2 (698)	74.0 (735)
2 Malignant neoplasms	(140–208)	87.9 (570)	80.0 (584)	79.1 (651)
3 Cerebrovascular diseases	(430–438)	25.5 (233)	24.1 (235)	26.0 (294)
4 Chronic obstructive pulmonary diseases	(490–496)	16.0 (120)	16.5 (136)	16.3 (149)
5 Motor vehicle accidents	(E810–E825)	13.7 (100)	14.3 (111)	13.2 (118)

Rates are per 100,000 population and are age-adjusted to 1940 US population (the second figure in each column gives the actual number of deaths in that period).

Source: http://hlunix.hl.state.ut.us/action2000/textdocs/uc.txt

Britain and the United States have collected information about death on a routine basis since the mid-nineteenth century. Although there are slight differences between Britain and the United States in the format of the death certificate and the system of recording deaths, the information provided is broadly similar. The medical practitioner who has dealt with the deceased provides information regarding the cause of death. This information is accompanied by date of birth, sex and occupational information relating to the deceased. This death certificate is incorporated into national mortality records and is eventually available for researchers to use in an anonymized format. In Britain and the United States, the death is also geo-referenced so that the area of residence of the deceased is known. Thus medical geographers and medical sociologists have a good record of where and when each death took place, and what caused it. Both Britain and the United States employ the ICD system of categorizing a cause of death (see Box 3.16).

In both Britain and the United States there is also a system in place for recording incidents of specific illnesses, called notifiable diseases. These range from certain infections which are more common in children, such as measles or meningitis, through to much rarer conditions such as Lassa fever. Certain types of food poisoning are also recorded and it is the statistics stemming from the

Box 3.17 A Severe Outbreak of Food Poisoning in Scotland

Sunday November 17 1996 Around 70 pensioners attend a lunch at Wishaw Old Parish Church, Lanarkshire in Scotland. They are served pre-cooked steak pies from the butcher John Barr & Sons.

Wednesday November 20 1996 Some who attended the lunch fall ill.

Thursday November 21 1996 The first pensioner who attended the lunch is rushed to hospital with food poisoning.

Friday November 22 1996 The number of pensioners in hospital grows. Lanarkshire Health Board issues a statement at 6 pm: 'It has become apparent that an outbreak of food poisoning has occurred in the Wishaw area.'

Saturday November 23 1996 There are 35 people at this stage reporting symptoms; 20 of them are in hospital. John Barr & Sons emerges as a possible source of the outbreak and cold meats are cleared from the shelves of what was the 'Scottish Butcher of the Year'.

Sunday November 24 1996 5 definite cases of E-coli 157 are admitted with another 4 giving hospital staff cause for concern.

Monday November 25 1996 Panic spreads through the local area. 42 patients are admitted to Monklands Hospital and 37 to Law Hospital. 6 adults and 1 child are seriously ill. The number of people with symptoms of E-coli rises to 68.

Tuesday November 26 1996 The first tragedy strikes – 80 year old Harry Shaw, an elder of Wishaw Old Parish Church, becomes the first fatality of the epidemic. 85 people have reported symptoms with 10 in a serious condition.

Wednesday November 27 1996 4 die on this day. Alex Gardiner (69), Jessie Rogerson (71), both from Wishaw, and Marian Muir (79) from Cleland and Nan Criggie from Bonnybridge bring the death toll to five. 107 people are now reporting symptoms.

Thursday November 28 1996 The gravy at the Old Parish Church is positively revealed as containing E-coli 157 – the first definite proof of the infectious source. 132 people show symptoms, with 49 people still in hospital.

Saturday November 30 1996 E-coli 157 is linked to a knife used in Barr's to cut raw meat and subsequently used to open bags containing cooked meat. The number of cases of E-coli rises to 117, with around 230 suspected.

Sunday December 1 1996 Monkland General Hospital closes its doors to GP admissions and opens a third ward to cope with rising number of E-coli cases. Suspected cases rise to 262.

Monday December 2 1996 280 cases across Scotland.

Tuesday December 3 1996 Moira Jackson, a 72 year old woman from the Wishaw area dies in Monkland Hospital, bringing the death count to six. Suspected cases rise to 307 with 168 confirmed.

Wednesday December 4 1996 Pensioner James Henderson (74) becomes the seventh to die.

Thursday December 5 1996 The Lord Advocate, Lord Mackay of Drumadoon, announces a Fatal Accident Inquiry.

Monday December 16 1996 Around 400 people are infected. John Barr has his shop windows smashed.

By **June 20 1997** the E-coli 157 epidemic had claimed its 20th victim.

Source: http://www.freelands.co.uk/e-coli.htm

Box 3.18 Cancer registries

Many countries of the world maintain cancer registries through which the incidence of different kinds of cancer may be tracked and monitored. The advent of the Internet has made many of these data readily accessible to researchers across the globe. Visit the website:

http://www.ikr.nl/canregs.htm

---

requirement to record such cases which play a key role when trying to track an outbreak. Many cases of milder food poisoning, causing diarrhoea, will pass fairly quickly and hence will not be reported to a doctor. However, food poisoning can sometime makes a person seriously ill. Box 3.17 presents a brief description of the Scotland's worst (recorded) outbreak of food poisoning, which took place in 1996. The notification of confirmed diagnoses provided by doctors was the key to controlling the outbreak.

As well as recording the incidence of certain infectious diseases, Britain and the United States (and many other countries – see Box 3.18) also record the instance of cancer diagnosis and these data form an important element in efforts to combat it. You can see data on cancer in America mapped, in Figure 3.6 later.

Finally, there are a host of data sets that record contact with health-care systems. General practitioners routinely record contact with their patients, including information about diagnosis or treatment. In addition, other data sets record admittance to hospital, the treatments that take place there and the outcome. Although these data sources have great potential as research tools, given that they record 'real' incidence of illness on a systematic basis, in practice they can be very much more difficult to access and to use than conventional survey data. In addition, they contain only information about people who were sick enough to need treatment, or who sought treatment. However, in an age of rapidly increasing computer power and the expanding automation of information recording systems we can expect the utility of these data sets to increase.

Analyzing data

So far in this chapter we have looked at what kind of information medical geographers and medical sociologists might be interested in, and then at the types of information that are readily available. Now we begin to think about the ways in which those data sets are manipulated and used in actual analyses. We will divide our brief look at this subject into three sections: *recoding variables, deriving indicators* and *statistical tests and models*. As mentioned before, it is well beyond the scope of this chapter to include all quantitative techniques; this section simply provides an introduction to some of them.

Recoding variables

Under this heading we include simplifications, adjustments and manipulations of raw data. This is carried out to make subsequent analyses more straightforward or more meaningful. One straightforward manipulation is to collapse the range of the responses to a given question into a limited number of categories. For example, we might ask people their occupation, but to use each as a separate category for analysis would mean that we might have thousands of categories, many with only one person in them. So we collapse this full range of occupations into a much smaller number of social class categories. For instance, if a person defines their job as a lawyer, that occupation may be reclassified as social class I; someone who says they work as a street cleaner is reclassified as social class V. Re-expressing raw data in this way means that while a lot of detail is necessarily lost, the subsequent data are much more manageable in terms of analysis. Other examples of categorizing variables include dichotomizing (breaking into two groups) continuous variables (which can have a range of values), such as height, weight or blood pressure. Variables can also be categorized into groups, such as actual age being put into an age group or health being described as 'very good', 'good', 'fair' or 'poor' (see Box 3.19).

It is important to remember that the recoding of raw data has an influence on the final result of the analysis. If a continuous variable is dichotomized into two categories, 'high' and 'low', then we have discarded a lot of information about the variation of that particular variable. However, in some circumstances converting continuous variables to discrete variables, or working with dichotomous variables, can give greater potential for the analysis of the relationship between that variable and others. Usually a compromise has to be made in terms of the balance of the detail which you might ideally want to include, and what is practicable in terms of data analysis. Be aware that such decisions about measurement and analysis are crucial. Similarly, knowing what is *not* included in an analysis, as well as what is included, is vital.

Deriving indicators

Deriving indicators refers to the conversion or combination of variables into a more complex indicator or index – using existing variables to build new ones.

Box 3.19 Terms used to describe variables

- **Continuous:** a continuous variable is one whose values can lie *anywhere* on a numerical scale. Continuous variables can have an infinite number of values along that scale. Common examples are height and weight.
- **Discrete:** a discrete variable is one whose values are limited to a finite number. Common examples are the number of cigarettes smoked per day, occupation and social class.
- **Category:** a category is one value within a discrete variable. Red, blue and green are categories of a discrete colour variable. Colour can also be continuous!

Box 3.20 Body Mass Index (BMI)

- BMI is simple, correlates to 'fatness', and applies to both men and women.
- To determine BMI, weight in kilograms is divided by height in metres squared.
- A BMI of below 17 is considered to be dangerously low, 17–20 is considered underweight, 20–25 is ideal, 25 to 29 is considered overweight and 30 or above is considered obese.

The indicator might describe a spatial area or a social group, or it might refer to a particular health outcome or to any aspect of life that is related to health. Some examples may help to make this more clear.

Box 3.21 Standardized mortality ratio (SMR)

What are SMRs?

The SMR is an indicator which tells us whether the mortality rate among a particular subgroup of a population is above or below the average for the whole population. Geographers typically use SMRs to show whether mortality rates are higher or lower than the national average in particular areas within a country. Sociologists often use SMRs to show whether mortality rates are higher or lower than average among particular types of people (e.g. different social classes).

How do I interpret an SMR?

If the SMR equals 100, the mortality rate among the subgroup is precisely the same as the wider population average. If it is below 100, the mortality rate is lower than average; if it is above 100 the mortality rate is higher than average. So, an SMR of 50 means the mortality rate is half the average, an SMR of 100 is average, and an SMR of 200 is twice the average.

How are SMRs calculated?

To calculate an SMR we need two numbers: (1) the number of deaths that took place amongst the subgroup and (2) the number of deaths we would expect to take place among that group, given the ages and sexes of the people in it.

Then we do a simple calculation (note that this is the indirect method of calculation):

$$\frac{\text{Number of deaths that took place}}{\text{Number of deaths expected}} \times 100$$

How do we know how many deaths to expect?

This is calculated by multiplying the number of people in each age and sex group by the average mortality rate for that age and sex group. So, if the mortality rate for a man aged 45–49 is 5 per 100 men per year, and there are 20 men of that age in the group, we would expect 1 of them to die in an average year. We add up all the expected deaths in each age and sex group to get a total figure.

Example 1 Body mass index (BMI) describes the relationship between height and weight in such a way as to identify those at the extremes of the balance between these two important physiological indicators. See Box 3.20 for more details.

Example 2 The standardized mortality ratio (referred to as the 'SMR') is an indicator of how the mortality rate in a particular area or among a particular group compares with a wider population average. The SMR is one of the most common indicators of mortality used in medical geography and medical sociology. Box 3.21 describes this in more detail and Research Example 1 at the end of this chapter gives an indication of how SMRs can be used to answer research questions.

Example 3 Deprivation scores (Box 3.22) are used to capture the extent of poverty and deprivation in a particular area, relative to a wider population or the rest of the country. They are usually derived from data describing the characteristics of the housing and population in an area. We can then look at the relationship between the level of poverty in an area and the health of the population who live there. Medical sociologists and medical geographers refer to this kind of data as *ecological* because it relates to features of the living environment or 'habitat'.

Box 3.22 Deprivation scores

What are they?
Deprivation scores are indices that attempt to describe the level of material poverty in an area. They are often used as an indicator of what life might be like for residents of that area or to suggest what the residents themselves might be like. The assumption is made that people living in a deprived area are often or usually, or are more likely to be, deprived individuals.

How are they calculated?
Deprivation scores are constructed by combining various indicators concerning the aggregate characteristics of an area's population, housing stock and socio-economic circumstances.

An example
The Townsend score is a commonly employed British deprivation index and combines measure of the unemployment rate of an area (indicating lack of material resources and job insecurity), overcrowded housing (indicating material living conditions), lack of owner occupied accommodation (a proxy indicator of wealth) and lack or car ownership (a proxy indicator of income). Data on each of these variables are standardized (so that they are numerically compatible) and combined together to give a single score. Geographers frequently make maps of deprivation by shading in bounded areas according to their deprivation score.

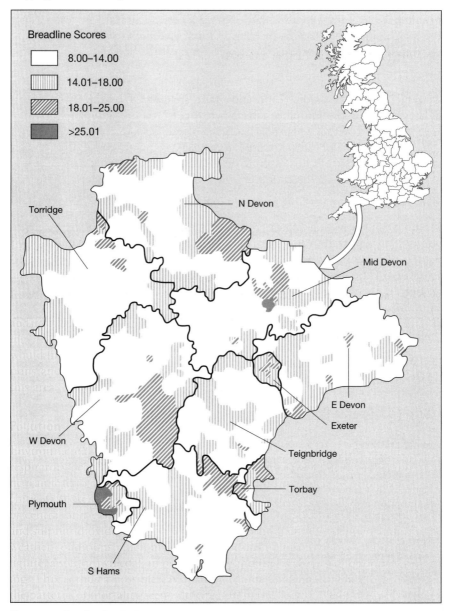

Figure 3.5 Deprivation in Devon.

Source: http://www.devon.gov.uk/dris/commstat/depr_mnu.html

Example 4 The Breadline Britain index is similar to a deprivation score but rather than giving a score for each area it estimates the proportion of households in an area that are below the poverty threshold, so a higher value indicates that the actual number of households living in poverty using this measure is higher. Figure 3.5 gives an example of this index mapped for a rural county of England.

Sometimes the construction of these indices marks the end of the data analysis and they themselves are the result of the research. More often, however, they form a building block used in further analysis.

Statistical tests

Various kinds of statistical test can be applied to the raw data, the recoded variables and the derived indicators that we have referred to above in order to investigate the relationship between variables. In quantitative medical geography and medical sociology statistical techniques are often used to seek to find out whether there is a relationship between different aspects of life and a health outcome. This is often done by testing an *hypothesis* (see Box 3.23).

There are a lot of commonly applied statistical procedures which it would be worth knowing about, but here we explore three of the most common or significant. (There are many statistics book available, but we particularly recommend Bryman and Cramer, 1990, and Rowntree, 1991 – see further reading, p. 84.)

Box 3.24 introduces the chi-square test, Box 3.25 introduces the concept of odds ratios and Box 3.26 explores multilevel modelling, a relatively new

---

Box 3.23 Hypotheses and falsification

A **hypothesis** is a statement about the relationship between variables that can be tested using statistical methods. For example, we might hypothesize that air pollution is related to asthma in children. In social science we usually test a null hypothesis, in this case it would be: air pollution is not related to asthma in children.

We test the null hypothesis rather than the hypothesis as western science is based on **falsification** – instead of seeking to prove that things are true, we seek to prove that they are probably not untrue!

Box 3.24 Common statistics: χ^2 (chi–square)

What is it?
The chi-square test is the most commonly used hypothesis test in the social sciences. It is a test of statistical significance, which refers to whether there is a relationship between two or more variables and whether this can be generalized to a population or if any relationship observed could be due to chance.

When can it be used?
This test can only be used for categorical and not for continuous data. For example, if you might look at whether there is a relationship between health outcome ('well' or 'ill') and wealth ('rich' or 'poor').

How does it work?
The chi-square test works on the simple principle that if there is no relationship between health and wealth then those who are 'well' and those who are 'ill' will be equally distributed between the categories 'rich' and 'poor'.

Box 3.25 Odds ratios

What are they?

Odds ratios are often used to describe the risk of an adverse health outcome which is associated with having a particular characteristic. The odds are expressed relative to a *reference* category.

Age group	Odds of poor health
0–15	1.0
16–44	1.5
45–64	2.0
65+	5.0

In this (hypothetical) example, the youngest age group is the reference category and hence has odds of 1.0. As we descend the table, the odds ratios rise (this pattern of rising risk is called a *gradient*). Those aged 45–64 are twice as likely as the *reference* category (the youngest group) to have poor health and those aged 65+ are five times as likely.

How do I calculate them?

Odds ratios can be calculated through a number of different statistical procedures ranging from simple cross-tabulation to more complex logistic regression.

Box 3.26 Multilevel modelling

What is it?

Multilevel modelling is a sophisticated type of statistical analysis which allows us to separate out the strength of influences at different spatial (or social) levels on an outcome. These can include the area in which we live.

It assumes that we live in a 'hierachy' of areas, for example a street sits within a neighbourhood, which sits within a city, which sits within a county and so on. This model also assumes that the characteristics of each of these areas may have an influence on health.

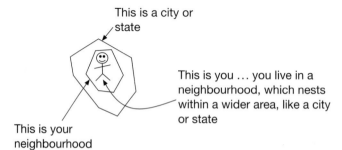

This is a city or state

This is you ... you live in a neighbourhood, which nests within a wider area, like a city or state

This is your neighbourhood

Multilevel models allow us to ask questions such as 'Which of these three things have the biggest influence on health: individual characteristics, neighbourhood characteristics or characteristics of your city or state?'

technique which can be very useful for connecting the relationships between individual characteristics, the characteristics of areas and health outcomes.

Section summary

Once data have been collected or obtained from a secondary source they can be recoded, converted into indices and used for analysis through statistical tests, or modelled. The complexity of the statistics and mathematics used in quantitative medical geography and medical sociology varies from the very simple to the very complex. In the twenty-first century, however, statistical software makes it easy to carry out complex statistical analyses on large data sets, and to do so very quickly. It is likely that the statistical power available to the researcher will far exceed their statistical knowledge! Always be sure that you understand the ways in which you manipulate your data and test your hypotheses, as the choice of techniques that can be used for analyzing the results have vital implications for their interpretation.

Mapping

Since this is a book about medical geography and many geographers draw maps to communicate their research findings and ideas, it is useful to understand something about the range of mapping techniques which are available to the medical geographer. It is also important to understand that maps are no longer just a way of presenting and summarizing information. The advent of geographic information systems (GIS) now permits the mapping process to be an integrated part of the research process. A computer user can use maps to interact with and to investigate data; GIS bring maps and their data 'alive'. Maps, or more particularly the spatial location of data, can be used to join items of information together, to search for patterns and as an interface to the statistical component of the research. This is not the place for a full discussion of how GIS work and what they are capable of, but it is important to be aware of the existence of these powerful tools (to learn more about GIS see: Burrough and McDonnell, 1998, and Martin, 1996).

Chloropleth maps

Figure 3.6 shows counties in the United States shaded according to their mortality rates from various forms of lung cancer. This is a chloropleth map, which entails shading areas of the map according to particular values. Showing data in this way can be very useful for observing general patterns and for seeing clusters of high or low values. However, this technique is not suitable for all research questions. Where the areas are largely unpopulated, or where the number of observations within each area is quite small, chloropleth maps can be misleading. The bigger areas on the maps are those that stand out most to the eye when reading the map, but these might not be the most important areas or contain the most people.

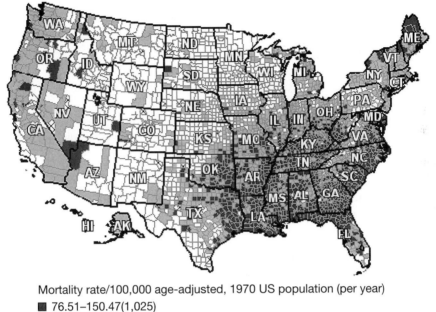

Mortality rate/100,000 age-adjusted, 1970 US population (per year)

- ■ 76.51–150.47(1,025)
- ▨ 62.08–76.51(994)
- ☐ 13.17–62.08(993)
- ▨ Sparse data(43)

Figure 3.6 Cancer in the United States.

Note: Number of countries shown in brackets.
Source: http://www-dceg.ims.nci.nih.gov/atlas/index.html

Cartograms

One way of dealing with chloropleth mapping problems is to use cartograms. A cartogram draws each area in proportion to the number of people, or observations, within it. Some cartograms use shapes, such as a circular dot, the size of which represents the population or value of the different areas being represented. You can see an example of this at the end of the chapter in Figures 3.9 and 3.10. Cartograms are also discussed extensively throughout Chapter 7. Figure 3.7 presents an area cartogram of the United States.

Point maps and boundaries

Where the incidence of the event or health outcome being mapped is very low, or where the spatial scale of analysis is very fine (perhaps just a few streets), it may be more appropriate to map using points rather than to shade in an area. This approach is quite often employed to view the geography of rare cancers, most notably in the detection of cancer clusters. One advantage of mapping points is that they may be grouped together in many different ways for analysis; drawing boundaries is an important aspect of medical geography. For example, Figure 3.8 shows the different ways that we can draw boundaries around a small number of

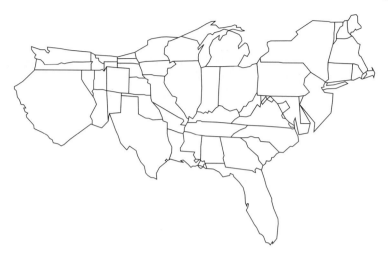

Figure 3.7 The United States with state boundaries redrawn to reflect population size.

Source: http://www-viz.tamu.edu/faculty/house/cartograms/1996Cartogram.html

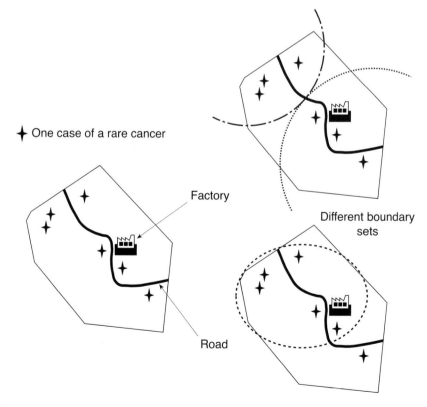

Figure 3.8 Comparing boundaries.

cancer cases, and the implications for analysis. Which of the alternative boundaries would lead you to suspect a cancer cluster around the factory? Or does the road look a more likely causal candidate (if indeed there is a candidate)? How much bigger would you like the extent of the map to be before you can be sure that this was indeed a cluster rather than just the normal incidence across the country? One particular advantage of GIS is their ability to draw boundaries such as the ones in Figure 3.8 many times over, with many different specifications and to carry out statistical tests automatically to determine whether there is indeed a genuine cluster of cases and to what extent this could be the product of chance alone. This allows the researcher to be sure that the results they have found are not just a function of the particular way in which the boundaries have been drawn.

Summary and research examples

We began this chapter by considering the types of information that are of interest to medical geographers and medical sociologists. We then explored various sources of information and the type of data they produce. Next we briefly considered the types of analysis we might wish to pursue using these data sources. At each point we have tried to focus on how medical geographers and medical sociologists think when they plan and carry out their research. Now we will present two specific examples of research that demonstrate some of the concepts and processes that have been presented in this chapter.

Research example 1

This example is drawn from our own research on the changing geography of mortality in Britain. We take this example further in Chapters 5 and 7. Here the example will be presented using the same terms which we have used throughout this chapter; we begin by outlining the research question.

Research question: How did the geographical pattern of mortality rates in Britain change between the early 1980s and the early 1990s and how much of that change can be accounted for by changes in the characteristics of the population?

Research approach: A relatively simple approach was adopted. SMRs (see Box 3.21) for each parliamentary constituency were calculated for the early 1980s and the early 1990s (a constituency is the area represented by one Member of Parliament in the House of Commons). The difference between the two SMRs was calculated to give the direction and magnitude of change in SMR for each constituency. The amount of that change which could be accounted for by changes in the socio-economic characteristics of the constituency population was then determined.

How is this research approach structured using the concepts introduced in this chapter?

Who are people? In this research we wanted to describe two types of information about the constituency populations: their demographic profile (in terms of age and sex) and their socio-economic characteristics (in terms of their social class structure and employment status). These characteristics were selected on the basis of our hypothesis that changes in the socio-economic characteristics of constituency populations could explain changes in their mortality rates. We therefore needed to know the demographic and socio-economic characteristics of the constituency populations at two points in time: the early 1980s and the early 1990s.

Where do people live? The research was concerned with mortality at the parliamentary constituency level (a constituency contains approximately 80,000 people). Our data source, the UK decennial censuses, told us about the population living in each parliamentary constituency.

What has happened to them? The health outcome in this research was death, but specifically deaths that occurred before the age of 65. Deaths before 65 are commonly referred to as 'premature deaths'. Age of death is recorded in mortality data, which derives from individual death certificates. Rates of death needed to generate the SMRs were drawn from published tables.

How were these data manipulated? The calculation of SMRs underpinned the entire research project. To answer the first question (how patterns of mortality have changed over time) SMRs were calculated for each constituency at two points in time. The two SMRs were evaluated by subtracting one from another to create an index of change. This index was mapped using a cartogram and the result is shown in Figure 3.9.

We next investigated how much of the pattern of this change could be explained (or 'accounted for') by the changing socio-economic characteristics of the constituency populations. As stated above and further examined in Chapter 4, the chance of premature mortality is strongly related to social class and employment status. If an area has a relatively high proportion of its population in lower social classes or in unemployment, we would expect the mortality rate in that area to be higher than the national average. Therefore, if between the early 1980s and the early 1990s a constituency experienced an increase in its unemployment rate or a change in the social class composition of its population, that might explain changes in its mortality rate. Our hypothesis was that these factors would explain the majority of change in mortality rates shown in Figure 3.9.

The hypothesis was tested by making the calculation of the SMR slightly more complex, to take account not only of the differences in mortality rates between different age/sex groups, but also of the different mortality rates of groups defined by age, sex, *social class and employment status*. By creating an SMR that takes account of social class and employment status and comparing it with an SMR based on age and sex alone, it was possible to determine how much of the change shown in Figure 3.9 was accounted for by changes in the social class and employment status composition of each constituency. The 'fit' between our hypothesis and the actual changes in mortality rate that took place is illustrated in Figure 3.10. In fact in 95 per cent of constituencies in Britain,

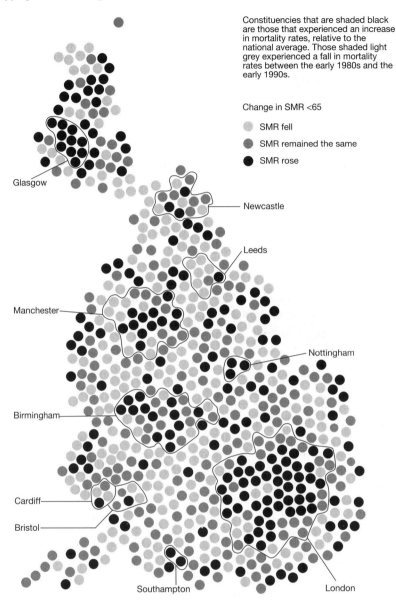

Constituencies that are shaded black
are those that experienced an increase
in mortality rates, relative to the
national average. Those shaded light
grey experienced a fall in mortality
rates between the early 1980s and the
early 1990s.

Change in SMR <65

○ SMR fell

● SMR remained the same

● SMR rose

Glasgow

Newcastle

Leeds

Manchester

Nottingham

Birmingham

Cardiff

Bristol

Southampton

London

Figure 3.9 Changes in death rate compared with the national average for parliamentary constituencies, early 1980s to early 1990s.

changes in the social class and employment status characteristics of the population account for changes in the constituency mortality rate to within 5 per cent.

More information about this piece of research can be found in Mitchell *et al.* (2000) *Inequalities in Life and Death: What if Britain Were More Equal?*

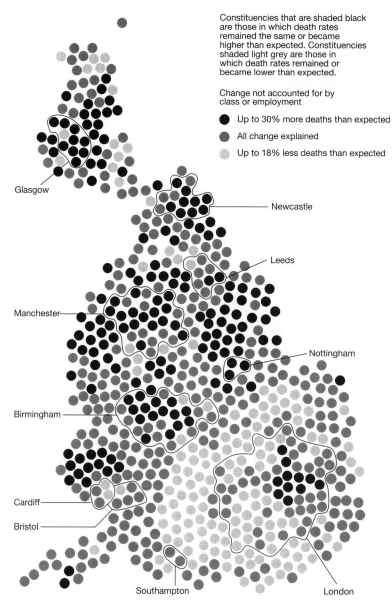

Constituencies that are shaded black
are those in which death rates
remained the same or became
higher than expected. Constituencies
shaded light grey are those in
which death rates remained or
became lower than expected.

Change not accounted for by
class or employment

● Up to 30% more deaths than expected

● All change explained

○ Up to 18% less deaths than expected

Glasgow

Newcastle

Leeds

Manchester

Nottingham

Birmingham

Cardiff

Bristol

Southampton

London

Figure 3.10 Explaining the change

Research example 2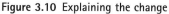

This research looks at the relationship between suicide and area-based measures
of deprivation and social fragmentation and is taken from research by Whitley
et al. (1999). It draws on a number of different kinds of data and analysis which
we have explored in this chapter.

81

Research question: Are the characteristics of an area (as measured by indices of deprivation and social fragmentation) associated with age-specific suicide rates?

Research approach: Two kinds of index which describe the nature of an area were calculated for parliamentary constituencies in Britain. One of these indices was the Townsend deprivation score (see Box 3.22) and the other was an index of social fragmentation (explained further below). Using the ICD codes (see Box 3.16) on mortality statistics, age- and sex-specific suicide rates were calculated for the constituencies. A statistical technique called regression was used to examine the strength of the association between suicide rates and the two measures of deprivation and social fragmentation.

How is this research approach structured using the concepts introduced in this chapter?

Who are people? In this research information about groups of people was captured in a derived index. The research used indices of deprivation and social fragmentation to characterize aspects of the nature of the population in question. This was an analysis of the relationship between a 'type of area' and the rates of suicide that occur there – an ecological study.

The Townsend deprivation index is derived from census data and gives each area a score based on: the percentage of economically active residents who are unemployed, the percentage of private households that do not possess a car, the percentage of private households not in owner occupied accommodation and the percentage of private households with more than one person per room.

Two different indices of social fragmentation were used: (1) average abstention rates in national elections between 1979 and 1992 and (2) an index derived from census data which included information on private renting, single person households (aged <65), unmarried persons and mobility in the previous year. This index is rather like a deprivation score in that it combines census data in a manner intended to capture some aspect of life in the area, in this case a lack of social connectedness or cohesion.

Where do people live? As explained above this research was based on British parliamentary constituencies.

What has happened to them? In this case the health outcome is cause-specific mortality: suicide. As described above specific causes of death are described by their ICD code and in this research the appropriate ICD codes were E950–E959 and E980–E989 (unexplained accidents were included).

What sources of data were used? Data about the electorate's response to an election were used in this research. This is an excellent example of the use of a data set which might not at first be thought applicable to health research. It is an illustration of the artificial boundaries that lie between different fields within social science. Censuses and mortality statistics formed the rest of the data set.

How were the data manipulated? The suicide rates for each age/sex group were calculated by working out the number of deaths from this cause relative to the size of the age/sex population group.

Research results: Higher abstention, social fragmentation and deprivation were associated with higher suicide rates in all age and sex groups, with the association being strongest for social fragmentation. When further work explored the changes in these indices and suicide rates over time it was discovered that increases in the social fragmentation index and in deprivation rates were also associated with increases in suicide rate across all age and sex groups. Since areas that have a high deprivation score tend to be the same as the ones with a higher degree of social fragmentation, statistical techniques were used to separate out the influence of these two characteristics. It was discovered that social fragmentation was the more important of the two.

Further thoughts: This research is an excellent example of the way in which medical geography and medical sociology fit together, and the ways in which information about area and about population can be amalgamated so that one may be used to make inference about the other. The authors of this study also issued an important warning:

> **It is important to recognize the limitations of ecological studies. Although socially fragmented areas have higher suicide rates, the people who commit suicide may not share the characteristics of the populations from which they are drawn. Moreover, the direction of the association is unclear, and it may be that people at high risk of suicide choose to live in socially fragmented areas or that these areas contain more hostels for mentally ill people. In addition, other factors may influence constituency level suicide rates, and the social fragmentation index may simply be a proxy for one or more of these.**

To learn more about this research read Whitley *et al.* (1999).

Conclusion

This chapter has focused on the ways in which medical geographers and medical sociologists think, the questions they pose, the data sets they use and the kinds of analyses they conduct. It was certainly not an exhaustive list of data and techniques used in this field, but it has nonetheless introduced some of the problems with, and potential solutions to, tackling sociological and geographical research questions about health in a quantitative way.

Almost all of the topics touched on in this chapter can be explored in more depth in the literature, both in academic journals and in other books, and increasingly on the Internet. Below are some suggested activities which may stimulate your interest further.

Further reading

- Wallace, D. and Wallace, R. (1988) *A Plague on Your Houses*. Verso: London.
  This book is part thriller, part textbook. It is easy to read and gives an excellent explanation of the principles of medical geography and medical sociology applied in an exciting real-world situation. The book focuses on the outbreak of house fires in New York between the 1970s and 1990s and the subsequent consequences in terms of

public health (with considerable reference to AIDS, drug abuse and crime). It is a gritty tale of the interface between politics and science.

- Denzin, N. and Lincoln, Y. (eds) (1994) *The Handbook of Qualitative Research*. Sage Publications: London.
  This book is a substantial (though expensive) resource which covers theoretical and practical issues concerning qualitative research in general.
- Pope, C. and Mays, N. (eds) (2000) *Qualitative Research in Health Care*. BMJ Publications: London.
  A useful and succinct book outlining the basics of the key qualitative methods currently employed in health-related research.
- Flowerdew, R. and Martin, D. (eds) (1997) *Methods in Human Geography: A Guide for Students Doing a Research Project*. Longman: Harlow.
  A practical text covering all stages of the research process which includes quantitative methods but also some very instructive chapters on qualitative methods, in terms of both data collection and data analysis.
- The details of the statistical methods and GIS books that we recommend are:
  Bryman, A. and Cramer, D. (1990) *Quantitative Data Analysis for Social Scientists*. Routledge: London.
  Rowntree, D. (1991) *Statistics Without Tears*. Penguin: London.
  Burrough, P. and McDonnell, R. (1998) *Principles of Geographical Information Systems*. Clarendon Press: London.
  Martin, D. (1996) *Geographic Information Systems: Socioeconomic applications*, 2nd edition. Routledge: London.

Suggested activities

- A film to watch: *Erin Brockovich*, starring Julia Roberts (directed by Steven Soderbergh, Universal Films, 2000).
  This entertaining film touches on issues of public health in relation to a particular source of pollution. Based on a true story, this is the tale of Erin Brockovich, a divorced working mother of three, who discovers that contaminated water is causing illness in people living in a certain area, and pursues the utility company responsible for the pollution for damages. This is in essence a classic medical geography or medical sociology issue: how to prove that a source of pollution is affecting the community.
- Find out what the most common cause of death in your neighbourhood is. Your local library may well carry the information you need to do this, and increasingly local government make these statistics available through their websites.
- Fill in the specimen death certificate as you think it might read for you (a slightly morbid exercise but certainly thought-provoking!).
- Surf to www.social-medicine.com and read about current research into health inequalities.

References

ASH (Action on Smoking and Health) (2000) *Basic Facts No. 2: Smoking and Disease* (www.ash.org.uk).

Bartley, M. (1994) Unemployment and ill health: understanding the relationship. *Journal of Epidemiology and Community Health*, 48: 333–7.

Bryman, A. and Cramer, D. (1990) *Quantitative Data Analysis for Social Scientists*. Routledge: London.

Burrough, P. and McDonnell, R. (1998) *Principles of Geographical Information Systems*. Clarendon Press: London.

Goldberg, D. and Williams, P. (1988) *A User's Guide to the General Health Questionnaire*. NFER-NELSON: Windsor.

Harrison, S. and Dourish, P. (1996) *Re-place-ing Space: the roles of place and space in collaborative systems*, Proceedings of ACM 1996 Conference on computer-supported cooperative work, November 16–20, 1996, Boston: USA.

High Times Magazine, 'Marijuana by the numbers', July 1999, New York.

Hillen, T., Schaub, R., Hiestermann, A., Kirschner, W. and Robra, B.-P. (2000) Self-rating of health is associated with stressful life events, social support and residency in East and West Berlin shortly after the fall of the wall. *Journal of Epidemiology and Community Health*, 54: 575–80.

Kerrison, S. and Macfarlane, A. (eds) (2000) *Official Health Statistics: An Unofficial Guide*. Arnold: London.

Kuh, D. and Ben-Shlomo, Y. (eds) (1997) *A Life Course Approach to Chronic Disease Epidemiology: Tracing the Origins of Ill-health from Early to Adult Life*. Oxford: Oxford Medical Publications.

Lee, A.J., Crombie, I.K., Smith, W.C.S. and Tunstall-Pedoe, H.D. (1991) Cigarette smoking and employment status. *Social Science and Medicine*, 33: 1309–12.

Martin, D. (1996) *Geographic Information Systems: Socioeconomic Applications*. 2nd edn, Routledge: London.

Mathers, C.D. (1995) *Health Differentials Among Australian Children*. Health Monitoring Series No. 3, Australian Institute of Health and Welfare: Canberra.

Mitchell, R., Dorling, D. and Shaw, M. (2000) *Inequalities in Life and Death: What if Britain Were More Equal?* The Policy Press: Bristol.

Morris, J.K., Cook, D.G. and Shaper, A.G. (1992) Non-employment and changes in smoking, drinking and body weight. *BMJ*, 304: 536–41.

Moser, K.A., Goldblatt. P.O., Fox, A.J. and Jones, D.R. (1987) Unemployment and mortality: comparison of the 1971 and 1981 longitudinal study census samples. *BMJ*, 294: 1353.

ONS (1997) *Mortality Statistics: General*. Series DH1 no. 28, The Stationery Office: London.

ONS (2000) *Living in Britain – Results from the 1998 General Household Survey 1998*. The Stationery Office: London.

Power, C. and Estaugh, V. (1990) Employment and drinking in early adulthood: a longitudinal perspective. *British Journal of Addiction*, 85: 487–94.

Rowntree, D. (1991) *Statistics Without Tears*. Penguin: London.

Shaw, M., Mitchell, R. and Dorling, D. (2000) Time for a smoke: one cigarette is equivalent to 11 minutes of life expectancy. *BMJ*, 320: 53.

Wald, N. (1991) *UK Smoking Statistics*, 2nd edn. Oxford University Press: Oxford.

Whitley, E., Gunnell, D., Dorling, D. and Davey Smith, G. (1999) Ecological study of social fragmentation, poverty, and suicide. *BMJ*, 319: 1034–7.

Wiencke, J.K., Thurston, S.W., Kelsey, K.T., Varkonyi, A., Wain, J.C., Mark, E.J. and Christiani, D.C. (1999) Early age at smoking initiation and tobacco carcinogen DNA damage in the lung. *Journal of the National Cancer Institute*, 91(7): 614–19.

Chapter 4

The social and spatial patterning of health

Chapter summary

In this chapter we begin to put some of the sociological and geographical tools covered in the first section of this book into practice and look at some of the evidence for the social and spatial patterning of disease in contemporary societies. We start by looking at the global picture to see to what extent health trends vary among countries. Next we look at particular regions of the world, considering how patterns of mortality have changed across central and eastern Europe and the possible explanations for this. We go on to consider differences in health at the regional level within countries, looking at the European Union and in particular Britain, and finish by considering the smaller spatial scale of local differences in health.

Introduction

In the previous chapter we reviewed some of the tools used by sociologists and geographers to study patterns and trends in health and illness. These included concepts to help us to organize our thinking, sources of data for addressing research questions, and ways of describing and analysing that data, such as mapping techniques and statistical methods. Here we look at the social and spatial patterning of disease at a number of geographical levels. At each geographical scale we look at how the patterns observed can be explained and consider the interaction of spatial factors with social factors. To what extent are the differences in life expectancy between countries explained by how wealthy those countries are? What role do behavioural factors such as smoking, diet and alcohol consumption play in explaining differences in health between different areas? Do men and women experience similar health chances in similar areas? Our main organizing theme is thus spatial, moving from the global to the local scale, but we shall also consider the extent to which health chances can vary by socio-economic indicators within each area, and by gender.

The global picture

The most reliable way in which to consider health variations across different nations is to look at mortality; for reasons discussed in Chapter 3 this is our best available indicator. From mortality data – knowing how many people die in a year, and their age and sex – we can calculate life expectancy (see Box 4.1). At the global scale there are significant differences in life expectancy between the different nations of the world (see Figure 4.1). The map shows how average life expectancy (in this map it is combined for men and women) varies across the globe. Life expectancy is highest in North America, western and northern Europe where it is now on average over 75 years, and lowest in Africa where in some countries it is below 40 years.

As you are probably aware, life expectancy is generally much lower in poorer countries than it is in the much richer industrialized countries. Those living in countries with what the United Nations terms 'high human development', which is measured by using indicators of education (such as literacy and enrolment rates) and adjusted real income (see Box 4.2) as well as life expectancy, can expect to live, on average, for 77 years. Those people living in areas with 'low human development' on the other hand can expect to live for only 50.6 years, whereas the population in areas of 'medium human development' has an average life expectancy of 66.6 years. There are thus substantial differences between the life chances of people living in different regions of the world. Notice, however, that there is a 16-year difference between low and medium development, and less than an 11-year difference between medium and high development. Look at Figure 4.2 and you will see this phenomenon in more detail.

The UN measure of human development is unusual in that it includes a range of indicators. Many people use the terms 'developed' and 'developing' when they really mean 'rich' or 'poor'. The terms 'developing' and 'developed' can be interpreted as having a moral overtone, implying that those countries that have 'developed' have 'done the right thing' and that the problems of the

---

Box 4.1 Life expectancy

Life expectancy refers to the years of life that a person or group can expect to live. It can be calculated from birth (giving total life expectancy) or from other ages: commonly ages 1 and 15. Life expectancy is a predictive or fictional concept in that it is based on the expectation of the average length of life assuming that current death rates continue. Life expectancy is calculated by using a life table. This is a summarizing technique used to describe the pattern of mortality and survival in a population. It tells us, out of an initial population (for example, 10,000 people), how many survive to each age, the proportion dying at each age (given age-specific death rates) and the life expectancy of those surviving to different ages. It also allows us to estimate the average life expectancy for those 10,000 people as a whole. As men and women have distinctive death rates, these life tables are calculated separately for each sex.

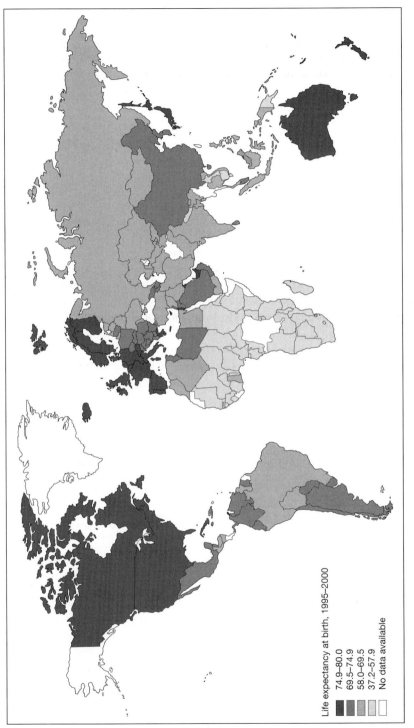

Life expectancy at birth, 1995–2000

- 74.9–80.0
- 69.5–74.9
- 58.0–69.5
- 37.2–57.9
- No data available

Figure 4.1 Life expectancy at birth across the globe, 1995–2000.

Source: Drawn by the authors from UN (2000).

Box 4.2 Gross domestic product (GDP)

GDP is the total value of the production of goods and services in a nation, measured over a year. Dividing by the number of people in the population gives the GDP per capita. GDP is the main indicator used to compare the income/standard of living in a country. However, it is an imperfect measure, as it does not include informal production or services, such as subsistence production or unpaid domestic work/activities.

poorer countries will disappear once they have 'developed'. Here we prefer to use the descriptors 'rich' and 'poor' instead.

Figure 4.2 shows that, as we have already noted, on the whole there is a relationship between the wealth of a country and the life expectancy of its inhabitants. However, this relationship is strongest for the poorer countries, with less than $5,000 GDP per capita per year, as Wilkinson (1996) has pointed out. Above this level increases in national wealth only seem to lead to relatively slight increases in life expectancy. We can use the statistical technique of correlation as a measure of the strength of association between two variables (see Box 4.3). In this case the correlation coefficients are as follows: for all countries $r = 0.67$, for

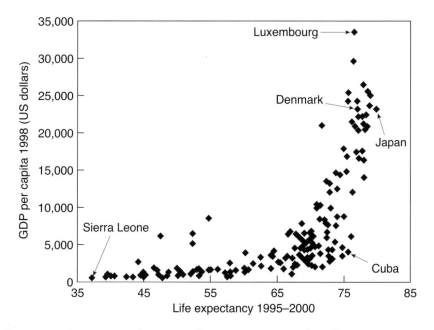

Figure 4.2 Life expectancy (1995–2000) and GDP per capita (1998) for countries of the world.

Note: Each point on the graph represents a country. The highest life expectancy = Japan; highest life expectancy under $5,000 = Cuba; lowest life expectancy = Sierra Leone; highest GDP = Luxembourg.

Source: Drawn from data in UN (2001).

Box 4.3 Correlation

If the change in the amount of one variable A is accompanied by a proportional change in the amount of another variable B, and that change in B does not occur if A does not change, then the two variables A and B are said to be correlated.

If an increase in A is associated with an increase in B then the two are said to be *positively* correlated. If an increase in A is associated with an decrease in B then the two are said to be *negatively* or *inversely* correlated.

An indicator of the strength of the relationship between two variables that are correlated is the *correlation coefficient* Pearson's r. This can vary from -1 to $+1$. When $r = 0$ there is no association between the two variables; when $r = -1$, there is said to be a *perfect negative* relationship; when $r = +1$ there is said to be a *perfect positive* relationship between the two variables.

When two variables are correlated but there is no causal link between them, then the correlation is said to be 'spurious'.

---

those under \$5,000 GDP per annum $r = 0.78$ and for those with more than \$5,000 $r = 0.63$. As you learn more about statistical techniques you will come to realize that far more complex statistics could be used here, the variables could be transformed and disaggregated further – however, we believe that this most simple analysis is most telling. The relationship is shown to be strongest for the poorer countries (see Figure 4.3). Wilkinson suggests that beyond a certain level of national wealth, other factors, such as the *distribution* of income within a country, are important in influencing population health, in addition to the amount of wealth that country produces. It is not only the *absolute* amount of wealth that is thus important to health, but also the amount of wealth people hold *relative* to others.

Causes of death across the world

There are other factors that distinguish the patterns of mortality in parts of the world with high and low average life expectancy. One of these is the causes of death which are most common. In Figure 4.4 two pie charts show the proportion of deaths from different causes for the rich and poor areas of the world in the late 1990s. In the richer areas of the world the category accounting for the highest proportion of deaths – 46 per cent – is circulatory diseases, with cancers accounting for 21 per cent of all deaths. By contrast in the poorer areas of the world the largest proportion of deaths are attributable to the category 'infectious and parasitic' diseases, which account for 43 per cent of all deaths. These two contrasting regions are places said to be before and after the *epidemiological transition*, which refers to the shift away from infectious diseases as the main cause of mortality in a society, as these are replaced by chronic, degenerative diseases, such as heart disease and cancer. The richest countries went through this transition in the early decades of the twentieth century (Wilkinson, 1996). Remember, however, that the notion of 'transition' may be spurious – it im-

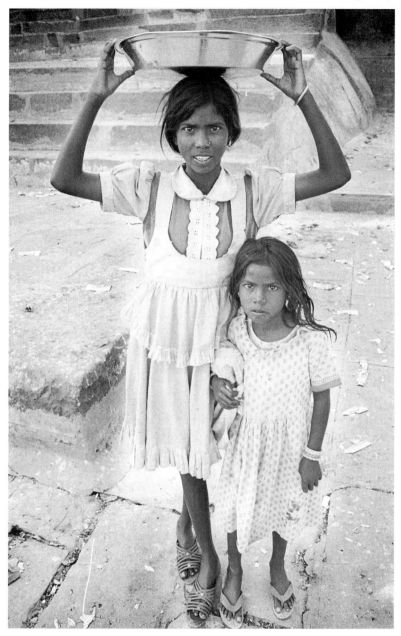

Figure 4.3 India, 2000.

Source: Photograph by Ben Joyner.

plicitly assumes that all countries are on the same trajectory and that the poor will catch up with the rich in time. There is little evidence of this happening to date. We shall return to the so-called 'diseases of affluence' later in the chapter.

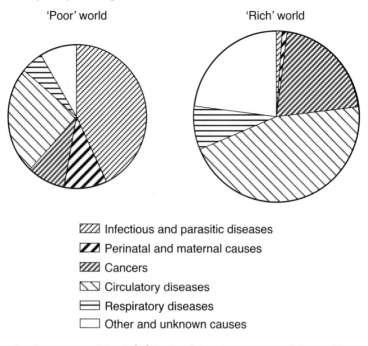

Figure 4.4 Leading causes of death (%) in the rich and poor areas of the world, 1997.

Note: The original source refers to the 'developed' and 'developing' world.
Source: WHO (1998b).

Much of the improvement in total life expectancy seen in the richer countries over the past century has been due to reductions in infant mortality rates. Similarly, it is babies and children who are most at risk from death from infectious diseases in the poorer countries. These infectious diseases are relatively few in number; five conditions account for most of the child mortality in poor countries: diarrhoea, acute respiratory infections, malaria, measles and perinatal conditions. Effective and inexpensive remedies, such as oral rehydration therapy for diarrhoeal disease, exist to deal with many of these conditions (see Box 4.4).

Box 4.4 A fair world?

- Every year more than 5 million people die from diarrhoeal diseases caused by water contamination.
- 840 million people worldwide are malnourished.
- The income of the richest fifth of the world's population is 74 times that of the poorest fifth.
- More than 880 million people lack access to health services.
- More than 250 million children are working as child labourers.

Source: UN (2000), p. 22.

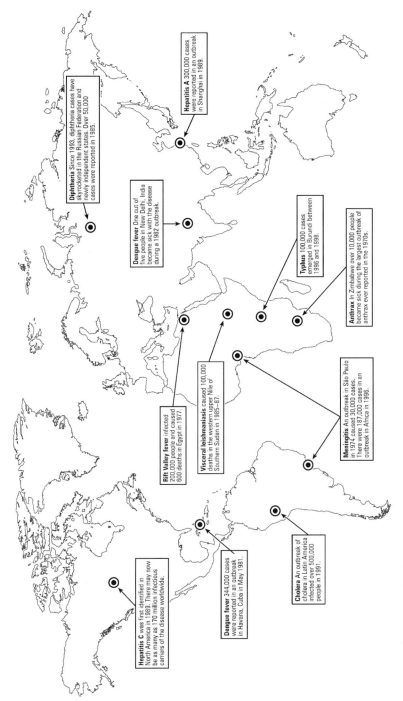

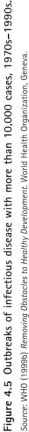

Figure 4.5 Outbreaks of infectious disease with more than 10,000 cases, 1970s–1990s.

Source: WHO (1999b) *Removing Obstacles to Healthy Development.* World Health Organization, Geneva.

Figure 4.5 shows large outbreaks of infectious diseases which occurred across the globe between the 1970s and 1990s. Note in which parts of the world these have tended to occur – many of these epidemics have been in Africa or South America. This map shows how infectious diseases are spread far more easily in conditions of poverty today. The same was true in the countries we now call developed in the recent past (just six to ten generations ago). However, a concentration of large outbreaks of disease can mask the importance of the persistent and much larger levels of poor health that occur constantly but not in such dramatic space/time clusters.

Some of the infectious diseases on the map in Figure 4.5 are diseases that we came across in the historical context of Chapter 2, such as cholera, and are what we might call 'old' infectious diseases. Other diseases that would fall into these categories are tuberculosis (TB, or 'consumption' as it used to be known), typhoid and plague. Tuberculosis was one of the main causes of death in Northern Europe and the Americas until about 1900. As living conditions improved and effective treatments were developed, the disease was virtually (but not completely) eliminated in those regions of the world. In the developing world, however, TB is still a leading killer, and it particularly affects young adults. In some developed countries in recent years rates of TB have either ceased to decline, or risen slightly, reflecting either rising poverty rates and/or immigration of infected groups. For example, Bhatti *et al.* (1995) report that despite steady falls in TB notification rates in England and Wales throughout the twentieth century there was an increase of 12 per cent between 1988 and 1992; however, in poor areas, the increase was 35 per cent. In the United States, rates of tuberculosis infection in the homeless have been found to be related to HIV infection (Moss *et al.*, 2000).

As well as having the 'old' infectious diseases to contend with, and for which there are in the main part effective (if not affordable) treatments available, 'new' infectious diseases are emerging. The most significant new infectious disease is AIDS (see Box 4.5).

Averages, variation and exceptions to the rule

You will have noticed that we have been using the term 'on average' a lot in this section (see Box 4.6). Averages are a very useful tool for summarizing data. However, at the same time they can hide important variations in the data. For example, 'exceptions to the general rule' are masked when averages are presented. Consider the case of Cuba. In Figure 4.2 above, of the countries with per capita GDP of less than $5,000, Cuba has the highest life expectancy, at 75.7 years. This is the same as average life expectancy in Denmark, although the GDP per capita in Cuba is $3,100 compared with Denmark where it is over 7 times greater, at $23,690. Clearly, it is not only how much wealth a country has that matters for health, but what is done with that wealth. Box 4.7 presents more information about health in Cuba.

Box 4.5 AIDS

What is AIDS?

Acquired immune deficiency syndrome (AIDS) is a condition resulting from infection with the human immunodeficiency virus (HIV). HIV destroys helper T cells, which means that the body's immune system is suppressed, reducing its defence against infection. A person who has the virus is referred to as 'HIV positive'.

How do you get it?

HIV is transmitted through bodily fluids and the main route of transmission is through sexual activity, either homosexual or heterosexual. The two other main routes of transmission are through infected blood or blood products (for example in blood transfusions or when sharing intravenous needles) and from a mother to her child (either while the fetus is in the uterus, during the birth, or through breast milk). Ordinary social contact with a person infected with HIV involves no risk of infection.

How many people in the world have HIV/AIDS?

In 2000, 36.1 million people were living with HIV/AIDS, 5.3 million people were newly infected with HIV and 3 million people died from AIDS. The total number of people who have died from AIDS since the beginning of the epidemic is 21.8 million (UNAIDS/WHO, 2000).

Social aspects of AIDS

AIDS, like many other diseases before it, has evoked many social and sociological responses. Instead of responding to people with AIDS as simply ill and therefore in need of care, there is often a response that is mediated by moral value judgements. One of the most erudite writers on this topic is Susan Sontag. Sontag (1990) has written about the metaphors that people attach to illnesses such as TB and cancer, and the way the people become stigmatized. She has also extended her analysis to the way we think about AIDS:

> In contrast to the soft death imputed to tuberculosis, AIDS, like cancer, leads to a hard death. The metaphorized illnesses that haunt the collective imagination are all hard deaths, or envisaged as such. Being deadly is not in itself enough to produce terror. It is not even necessary, as in the puzzling case of leprosy, perhaps the most stigmatised of all diseases, although rarely fatal and extremely difficult to transmit. Cancer is more feared than heart disease, although someone who has had a coronary is more likely to die of heart disease in the next few years than someone who has cancer is likely to die of cancer. (Sontag, 1990, p. 126)

Mortality by age

Averages such as life expectancy also mask the age distribution of mortality within a population. A mean is disproportionately affected by extreme values, be they high or low, in a distribution. Average life expectancy is thus affected to a great extent by infant mortality. A country with a low average life expectancy is likely to have high rates of infant mortality. However, those who survive beyond the first year of life, and beyond childhood, will have a life expectancy higher than the 'average'.

Box 4.6 Averages

- **Averages** – are an extremely useful way of summarizing a large amount of data with one statistic. Averages can also be referred to as 'measures of central tendency'.
- **Mode** – this is the value that occurs most frequently in a set of data. A distribution can have more than one mode – if it has two modes it is referred to as bimodal, if it has more than two modes it is multimodal.
- **Median** – the median refers to the mid-point of a distribution. If all values are ordered in terms of magnitude, the one in the middle is the median
- **Mean** – this is what people usually mean when they refer to an average, and they are usually referring to the arithmetic mean. The arithmetic mean is equal to the sum of all the observed values divided by the total number of observations. The mean is very sensitive to extreme values, known as 'outliers'.

Let's look more closely at some mortality figures. Table 4.1 shows the age- and sex-specific mortality rates for Canada and Chile in 1994. For both countries the first year of life is relatively dangerous, and more so for boys than for girls. Death rates are then low in childhood and rise slowly from early adulthood and more quickly from later adulthood. The last column shows the ratio of these age-specific death rates in Chile compared with Canada. This reveals that the difference between the two countries is greatest in early life, thereafter their mortality profiles, at least by age, are more similar. Much of this difference in infant and child mortality will be accounted for by infectious diseases.

Box 4.7 Health in Cuba

Cuba's government guarantees free medical care for all, and there is one doctor for every 260 Cubans. All services are free and widely available. Many transmissible diseases have been eradicated through a massive vaccination programme.

However, the health system in Cuba is currently seriously affected by a lack of medicines and supplies due to the US embargo. Many traditional folk medicines have been used when modern medicines cannot be obtained.

	Cuba	Latin America
Life expectancy	75.4	68
Infant mortality	7.9/1,000 births	38/1,000
Under 5 mortality	12/1,000 births	47/1,000
Maternal mortality	21/1,000 births	178/1,000
Access to health services	98% population	73% population

Figures are for 1994.

Source: American Association for World Health (1997).

Table 4.1 Age- and sex-specific mortality rates and rate ratios per 100,000 (infant death rates per 100,000 live births) all causes, for Canada and Chile, 1994

Age	Canada		Chile		Rate ratio Chile : Canada	
	Male	Female	Male	Female	Male	Female
0	693.8	557.9	1,286.2	1,108.5	1.9:1	2.0:1
1–4	35.2	28.5	65.8	46.0	1.9:1	1.6:1
5–14	21.3	15.2	31.9	21.9	1.5:1	1.4:1
15–24	93.3	32.6	115.2	36.2	1.2:1	1.1:1
25–34	118.4	44.1	181.1	53.1	1.5:1	1.2:1
35–44	196.3	97.9	264.3	131.4	1.3:1	1.3:1
45–54	396.0	249.6	614.9	342.9	1.6:1	1.4:1
55–64	1,165.9	661.0	1,492.9	836.0	1.3:1	1.3:1
65–74	2,972.8	1,643.3	3,674.6	2,026.6	1.2:1	1.2:1
75+	9,262.9	6,845.9	10,745.4	8,042.0	1.2:1	1.2:1

Source: WHO (1998a).

It is reductions in rates of infant mortality that account for much of the overall improvement in life expectancy that rich countries have enjoyed. However, within the richer, industrialized nations there are still clear socio-economic gradients apparent in rates of infant, and child, mortality.

Figure 4.6 shows the dramatic decreases in infant mortality that have occurred in England and Wales since the early 1900s after relative stability in the latter part of the nineteenth century. The fall is quite staggering. How much lower can this rate get?

However, despite these absolute falls in rates there is still a clear social class gradient in infant and child mortality rates in England and Wales. Table 4.2 shows neonatal, postneonatal and infant mortality rates for the period 1993–95. Neonatal deaths (in the first 28 days after birth) tend to be from factors related to birth, such as being born prematurely; postneonatal deaths are more likely to be the result of external causes. From this table we can see that there are clear social class gradients in all three of these rates. Here the Registrar General's social class definition is used, which is based on occupation (see Box 4.8). Babies whose fathers work in jobs that are classified as 'professional' are more likely to survive the first year of life than those in 'semi-professional' occupations, and much more likely to survive than those whose fathers are unskilled manual workers.

Looking at deaths of older children, where the absolute numbers of deaths are even lower, even when we focus on one particular cause of death these social class gradients are again apparent – indicating the persistence and predominance of the effect of social class. Two researchers, Roberts and Power (1996) looked at child deaths from injury and poisoning in England and Wales around the years 1981 and 1991. These are the causes of death that are now most likely to kill children in this setting. Roberts and Power report that in 1981 the injury death rate for children in social class V was 3.5 times that of children in social

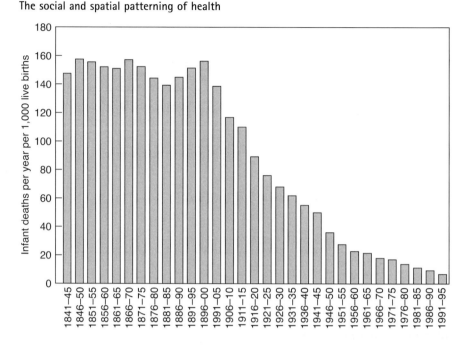

Figure 4.6 Infant mortality in England and Wales, 1841–1995.

Source: Drawn from ONS data (1997). © Crown Copyright 2000.

class I. By 1991 the rates for children in social class V were 5.0 times higher. This gap has widened because, although the rates for children of all backgrounds fell during the study period, they fell most for children whose parents worked in professional and non-manual occupations.

Table 4.2 Infant mortality rates by father's social class, England and Wales, 1993–95

Father's social class	Neonatal rate	Postneonatal rate	Infant rate
I	3.1	1.3	4.5
II	3.5	1.3	4.8
IIIN	3.9	1.6	5.5
IIIM	4.1	1.8	5.9
IV	4.6	2.0	6.6
V	4.9	2.8	7.7
England and Wales	4.1	1.8	5.9

Neonatal rate: number of deaths of babies under 28 days per 1,000 live births.

Postneonatal rate: number of deaths of babies aged 28 days and over but under 1 year per 1,000 live births

Infant rate: number of deaths of babies under 1 year per 1,000 live births.

Source: Botting (1997).

Box 4.8 Registrar General's social class (based on occupation)

Social class	Occupation type
I	Professional (e.g. accountant, electronic engineers)
II	Managerial and technical/intermediate (e.g. proprietors and managers – sales, production, works and maintenance managers)
IIIN	Skilled non-manual (e.g. clerks and cashiers – not retail)
IIIM	Skilled manual (e.g. drivers of road goods vehicles, metal working production fitters)
IV	Partly skilled (e.g. storekeepers and warehousemen, machine tool operators)
V	Unskilled (e.g. building and civil engineering labourers, cleaners, etc.)

Source: Bunting (1997).

Mortality: men and women

In many ways it is useful to have one statistic to refer to the life chances of a nation. However, this hides a very important difference between men and women. Women live longer, on average, than do men (see Table 4.3).

The life expectancy gap between men and women is larger in the richer countries of the world, and in those places the difference has become greater over time. For example, in England and Wales, the life expectancy gap between men and women was two years in the 1840s, but by the 1990s it was over five years (ONS, 1997).

Some of the improvement in female life expectancy can be accounted for by reduced maternal mortality – the death of a woman while pregnant or within 42 days of termination of pregnancy, regardless of the site or duration of pregnancy, from any cause related to or aggravated by the pregnancy or its management (WHO, 1999a). The five major causes are: haemorrhage (severe bleeding), sepsis (where bacteria cause decomposition), eclampsia (convulsions caused by

Table 4.3 Life expectancy for men and women

Level of 'human development' (UN indicator)	Men	Women	Difference
High	73.7	80.2	6.5
Medium	64.8	68.7	3.9
Low	49.7	51.5	1.8

Source: UN (2000).

Box 4.9 Maternal mortality in the world today

- Worldwide, nearly 600,000 women die each year as a result of complications arising from pregnancy and childbirth.
- For every woman who dies, many more suffer from serious conditions that can affect them for the rest of their lives.
- It is estimated that 5 million infant deaths per year are largely the result of poor maternal health and hygiene, inadequate care, inefficient management of delivery, and lack of essential care of the newborn.

Source: WHO (1999).

---

high blood pressure), obstructed labour and complications of unsafe abortion. Box 4.9 presents some sobering facts on maternal mortality.

In rich countries, maternal deaths have become increasingly rare since the 1940s – 1 in 4,000 women die from pregnancy-related problems; in some poor countries the rate is 1 in 12. This is one of the starkest measures differentiating the rich and poor world. Maternal deaths are a persistent feature of poor countries, and within those countries it is the poorest, most disadvantaged and least powerful who are most at risk.

One of the fundamental determinants of maternal mortality is the low social status of women, limiting their access to economic resources and basic education, which in turn affects their ability to make decisions about their health and nutrition. Cultural practices in some societies mean that women are secluded and denied access to care. Excessive physical work and poor nutrition, before and during pregnancy, are also contributing factors to poor maternal outcomes. Lack of access to essential obstetrical services is also a crucial factor, and is especially a problem for women in remote rural areas, or where there is little transport (see Box 4.10).

Section summary

In this first section we have taken a predominantly global perspective, looking at how health differs across various parts of the world. We have seen that there are very different life chances and causes of death that are responsible for the burden of mortality in the rich compared with the poor world. Taking this broad geographical view we have also learnt about some of the social dimensions to health, such as the importance of looking at different age-groups, and the different life chances of men and women. We have also seen the important role played by socio-economic factors – whether at the country level and considering life expectancy and GDP, or whether looking at infant mortality and social class in England and Wales, those who live in better off areas or who are in better off groups tend to have better health outcomes. We shall see more evidence of this later in the chapter.

Box 4.10 Cultural attitudes towards fertility and childbirth (Patel, 1994)

In the village of Mogra, in Rajasthan, India, childbirth is seen as the responsibility not only of the pregnant women, but of the entire household. Community resources are also pooled in order to ensure successful childbirth. Pregnancy and childbirth are considered normal and desirable for young women. As pregnancy is not considered a special condition, women are not generally given any concessions from physical work, and only at the last stage of pregnancy are they dissuaded from lifting heavy loads. Indeed, it is believed that regular physical activity aids labour and makes it less painful.

Because pregnancy is valued the pregnant woman's intake of food increases, and food cravings are indulged – for non-pregnant women food consists of an austere diet of certain staples. A determined effort is made by family and friends to satisfy a woman's cravings, which are considered to be partly the cravings of the unborn child. Food cravings that are not satisfied are thought to be expressed by the infant child, for example, by frequent dribbling. The nature of food cravings is thought to indicate the sex of the baby, sweet for a son and sour for a daughter.

Men are excluded from any participation in childbirth. Birth is attended by an experienced female relative or neighbour who provides comfort, support and reassurance; professionally trained nurses are rarely summoned. Modern medicine is rarely resorted to, usually only when the woman's life is in danger.

It is not expected that a woman will express pain during childbirth; groaning and screaming are disapproved of. As Patel says of a woman in labour:

> She rarely writhes in pain all by herself. She is the centre of attention for all those present beside her in the privacy of the room. They all involve themselves intensely with her. Their frisky movements, pauses, sounds, talk and facial expressions are in accordance with the woman's rhythm of pain, and give her much-needed strength and encouragement. Their serious participation in the process indicates that the child is desired by them collectively and that the mother is performing a heroic personal as well as social ordeal. The people around provide mechanisms that effectively prevent the labouring woman from turning hysterical or even losing her calm. The warmth of collective participation and emotional care is in sharp contrast to that experienced by labouring women in British hospitals which affect them adversely. (Patel, 1994, p. 117)

Fear and anxiety are thus not associated with childbirth in this setting. By the time a woman has her third child she will often give birth alone, at home, or even in the fields.

Comparing countries

In this section we focus in on comparing life chances in different countries. Such macro-level comparisons are useful because often the main source of variation is between countries rather than within them. However, where countries are of similar levels of affluence then within-country comparisons can usually tell us more. In this section we look in detail at a particular case study, considering recent trends in life expectancy in some of the countries of central and eastern Europe and the possible explanations that researchers have proposed for these trends.

Recent mortality trends in eastern and central Europe

the transition to market economies [in the region] is the biggest ... killer we have seen in the 20th century, if you take out famines and wars. The sudden shock and what it did to the system ... has effectively meant that 5 million [Russian men's] lives have been lost in the 1990s.

Omar Noman, in *BMJ* (1999) 319: 468.

Life expectancy is currently higher in western Europe than in central and eastern Europe, but this has not always been the case; this difference has largely emerged since the early 1970s. Since then, while average life expectancy has been steadily increasing in the West, it has been stagnating or even falling in some of the countries of central and eastern Europe. By the late 1990s the difference between these regions was substantial – greater than ten years. The map in Figure 4.7 shows the extent of the gap in the late 1990s, with the western European countries having the highest life expectancy, central Europe somewhere in the middle, and the countries of eastern Europe – in particular Russia, Ukraine and Belarus – experiencing the lowest life expectancy.

In the Soviet Union life expectancy began a steady decline in the mid-1960s which was sustained until 1991, when the decline increased. Between 1991 and 1994 life expectancy at birth for people of the countries of the former Soviet Union fell by four years for men and by 2.3 years for women. However, as we have noted above, averages can be a powerful summarizing tool, but can mask important detail. In this case, the increases in mortality rates were concentrated in the 35–44 year age group, where for men in 1995 mortality rates were four times higher than in western Europe (McKee, 2001).

The scale of the life expectancy crisis in Russia in the early 1990s is shown by the following quote from Bennett *et al.* (1998):

It is estimated that between 1990 and 1995 between 1.3 and 1.6 million premature deaths occurred in Russia. This compares to 55,000 Americans lost during the Vietnam war and 240,000 Americans dying from AIDS during the same period.

Figure 4.8 shows that in these four countries of the former Soviet Union life expectancy for women has been stable, with some slight declines over the 20 years from 1980 to 2000. For men, however, small increases have been followed by slight decline in the late 1980s, with further decline persisting into the 1990s; the decline for Russian men is particularly marked.

This situation of falling life expectancy is without precedent in modern history – in peacetime, and until the AIDS epidemic took hold, there was nowhere that health had declined to such an extent. This trend was seen as one of the most important public health issues at the end of the twentieth century. Looking at these trends more closely, by age, sex, cause of death, socio-economic group and geographical area gives us clues as to their possible cause. But note that this is an area of research that is current and developing, there are no hard

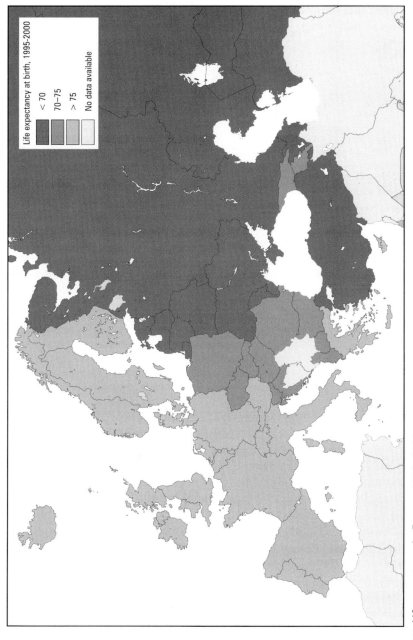

Figure 4.7 Life expectancy in Europe, 1995–2000.
Source: Drawn from UN data (2000).

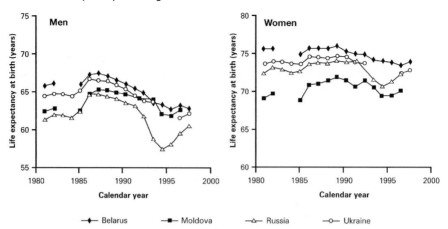

Figure 4.8 Trends in life expectancy for males and females at birth in four countries of the former Soviet Union, 1981–97.

Source: Redrawn from McKee (2001).

and fast answers or explanations; indeed the trends themselves are also changing. In addition, much of the data from this region are not as reliable as we would like them to be. However, we shall explore some of the possible explanations and the evidence for those explanations given the state of knowledge in this area. So what are these potential explanatory factors?

Pollution

Environmental pollution undoubtedly has an effect upon health, specifically on respiratory health. Pollution from heavy industry, as well as emissions from traffic, can lead to and exacerbate a number of conditions such as asthma and bronchitis. Children are particularly vulnerable. It is also established that the region of central and eastern Europe is a highly polluted area – levels of particulates and sulphur dioxide are 2–3 times the WHO air quality guidelines, and in some weather conditions much higher. Much of this pollution derives from the use of lignite, a soft brown coal, in power plants and this is also used for domestic heating. This is thus a possible candidate (an independent variable) for explaining the patterns of mortality seen in the region in the last couple of decades (see Box 4.11 for an explanation of dependent and independent variables).

So what is the impact of the high rates of pollution in particular parts of Europe on mortality? This is a very difficult area to research as it is very difficult to measure exposure levels, and it is also difficult to single out the effects of pollution. However, studies have tried to look at this by comparing the known 'dose–response' effect (see Box 4.12) of pollutants on health with the outputs of those pollutants, asking: is health worse where pollution is highest? One such study looked at the Czech Republic, where recent trends in mortality have been similar to, though less marked than, those in the countries of the former Soviet

Box 4.11 Dependent and independent variables

Within a particular study the dependent variable is the variable that we are aiming to explain; the variations in the dependent variable are said to be brought about by the independent variables(s). The variations in the independent variable are said to result in variations in the dependent variable. For example, an increase in traffic speed (independent variable) may lead to an increase in the incidence of fatal road traffic accidents (dependent variable). Another way to think of this is to consider the independent variables as the 'cause' and the dependent variable as the 'effect'. Whether a particular variable is considered to be independent or dependent is determined by the conceptual model of that particular study. For example, if we are seeking to explain the variation in crime rates between different areas we may have unemployment rates as one of our independent variables. Alternatively, we may be aiming to explain variations in unemployment rates themselves, making that the dependent variable.

In the example of falling life expectancy in central and eastern Europe (see text) the dependent variable is mortality, and the independent variables include pollution, the provision of health services, behavioural factors such as smoking, and socio-economic factors such as unemployment.

Union (see Bobak and Marmot, 1996). The research suggests that in the Czech Republic only 2–3 per cent of the total mortality was the result of pollution. Interestingly, this is similar to an estimate for the United States, where it has been suggested that 2 per cent of all mortality is attributable to environmental pollution.

It thus seems that while pollution may play a role, it is unlikely to be the main culprit. That there are other more important factors producing the reduction in life expectancy is also suggested by the fact that the areas within countries with the highest levels of air pollution are not those with the highest mortality. The area shaded in Figure 4.9, called the 'black triangle', is known to be the most polluted zone of the region, perhaps the most polluted region in the world. Comparing this to Figure 4.7 above illustrates that it does not coincide with the areas of lowest life expectancy.

Also, the recent fall in life expectancy has been most marked for men, particularly in the age-range of 35–44. Why should pollution have affected men so

Box 4.12 A 'dose–response' effect

A dose–response effect refers to the relationship observed between an independent and a dependent variable – the greater the dose of the independent variable, the greater the effect on the dependent variable. For example, the more toxins you inhale or ingest, the greater the detrimental effect upon your health, or the more alcohol you drink, the more intoxicated you will become. Dose–response relationships are sometimes taken as evidence for a causal link between variables.

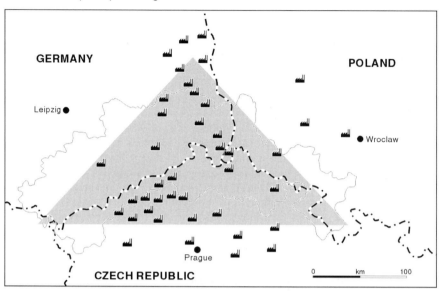

Figure 4.9 The 'black triangle' of pollution in central Europe.

much more than women? It was not just men in hazardous occupations for whom mortality rates reached a peak. Also, it is usually the respiratory health of the very young, and also the elderly, that is most affected by pollution, not those in mid-life. Thus while pollution in the region of central and eastern Europe is undoubt-edly at very high levels and may indeed be the cause of much morbidity, particularly respiratory illness, on closer investigation it appears to play a minor role in the decline in life expectancy that we are seeking to understand here.

The collapse of health services

Could the collapse of health services be a factor to consider? Perhaps it is prob-lems in the provision of health care that are leading to unnecessary premature deaths. All the former communist states aimed to provide free health care to all citizens ('free' in this instance meaning free at the point of delivery and funded through the central state – see Curtis and Taket, 1996, for a fuller discussion of different models of health service provision). In states such as the Soviet Union where prior to communism health care had been available only to a privileged few, the health service provided a basic 'no-frills' service which up to the 1970s was central in producing a decline in infectious diseases. However, the system increasingly suffered from a shortage of modern equipment, supplies and drugs. Clinics and hospitals were often overcrowded with poor standards of hygiene. Although the ideology of the system was one of fairness and accessibility to all, in reality the provision of services was skewed towards the large hospitals of the cities, at the expense of rural areas where often the staff would have low levels of training. While the service was ostensibly 'free', bribes or 'gifts' to medical personnel were commonplace, so that those with the most resources, or with political power or connections, would receive better care. After the collapse of communism the problems of health-care provision have become more acute, with a desperate lack of resources and supplies. Once again, the system privileges those who are able to pay.

Did this produce the fall in life expectancy observed? Clearly, the provision of health care in central and eastern Europe is currently in a state of crisis and is not what it could be (though it is better than in other parts of the world, it just depends what we are comparing it to). Inadequate care may have contributed to some of the deaths of individuals, but a large part of the mortality gap is unlikely to be attributable to the lack of medical care. Only some of the causes of death that make up a large proportion of the fall in life expectancy (see Table 4.4) are those that can be substantially reduced by the intervention of health care. For example, by the time people with cardiovascular (heart) disease seek medical treatment their condition is often acute and treatment may be palliative (giving relief from symptoms but not curing them) rather than curative. Also, 'external' causes of death, which include accidents, suicide and homicide, account for nearly a quarter of the life expectancy difference (1.41 of a total of 6.06 years). These are often deaths that even the most sophisticated health service cannot prevent. Thus while health-care provision may have been inadequate, it can be argued that it is not the main explanatory factor in this case.

We saw through the historical perspective in Chapter 2 that it is not just the medical system of a society that affects the general level of life expectancy. Rather we need to take a much wider perspective of the structure of society – the material conditions of living, the distribution of resources and a range of social factors. We shall consider such issues in this context below, but first we turn our attention to behavioural factors.

Table 4.4 Contribution to the gap in life expectancy between central and eastern Europe (including the former Soviet Union) and rest of the European region by age and cause of death, men and women combined, in 1993. Figures are difference in years (West minus East)

Cause of death	Age-group (years)				
	<1	1–34	35–64	65+	All ages
Infectious and parasitic diseases	0.30	0.10	0.08	−0.01	0.47
Cancer	0	0.05	0.25	−0.35	−0.05
Cardiovascular diseases	0	0.07	1.36	1.85	3.28
Respiratory disease	0.68	0.20	0.15	−0.05	0.97
Digestive diseases	0.02	0.03	0.08	−0.04	0.09
External causes (incl. accidents, homicide and suicide)	0.04	0.64	0.71	0.03	1.41
Ill-defined conditions	−0.10	0.01	0.04	0.18	0.12
Other diseases	0	0	−0.02	−0.20	−0.22
All causes	0.93	1.09	2.63	1.40	6.06

Source: Bobak and Marmot (1996).

'Unhealthy' behaviours – smoking, alcohol and diet

Perhaps the independent variables that we should be focusing on here are lifestyle factors, such as smoking, excessive alcohol consumption, poor diet and lack of exercise? These have all been shown to be related to poorer health outcomes. One group of researchers (Kubik *et al.*, 1995) report that cigarette sales increased dramatically through the 1960s and 1970s, and that between 1965 and 1989 the number of imported cigarettes doubled to 73 billion per year; in 1992 the adult smoking rate in Russia was 67 per cent. While rates of smoking have been decreasing in the West they have been increasing in the East. Interestingly though, while rates of cardiovascular diseases account for approximately half of the life expectancy gap between East and West, the East actually has a slight advantage in terms of cancer deaths. It is also hard to understand how smoking rates, which are consistently high in the East can account for a sudden rise in mortality rates as seen between 1991 and 1994 and the subsequent improvement, especially as many smoking-related illnesses have a long latency period.

In relation to diet, there is very little reliable, detailed evidence that can be used to compare the consumption patterns in eastern and western Europe. For example, some studies have found that fat consumption levels are fairly similar, although they do not have information on the type of fats consumed (saturated or unsaturated). However, the evidence does seem to suggest that, on the whole, diets in eastern Europe may contain more fat and less fresh fruit and vegetables than in the West.

However, by far the most attention in the issue of lifestyles and patterns of mortality in this region has been paid to the question of alcohol consumption. This is because the age-specific and cause-specific pattern of mortality, and the short-term fluctuations in rates, strongly point in this direction. This is supported by the fact that death rates from certain causes, such as cirrhosis and external causes, fell during 1985–86 (Leon *et al.*, 1997). It was during this period that President Gorbachev enforced an anti-alcohol campaign. State restrictions were placed on the supply and sale of alcohol, which initially had the effect of reducing consumption, but by the end of the 1980s home brewing had increased dramatically. In the early 1990s restrictions were lifted and with an increase in real wages the relative cost of alcohol fell.

Table 4.5 shows cause-specific death rates for 1984, 1987 and 1994 in Russia. When the authors of this study looked more closely at the patterns by age, sex and cause of death, they found three patterns which hold for all causes, apart from cancers:

1 For ages 20–69, rates decreased between 1984 and 1987 and increased between 1987 and 1994.
2 The largest increases were observed in the age range 20–45, whereas there were very small changes for infancy, childhood and old age.
3 Men and women showed very similar *relative* increases and decreases, even though the *absolute* mortality rates for women were much lower.

Table 4.5 Age-standardized (to European population) mortality rates per million for Russia by sex, year and cause

	1984		1987		1994	
	Male	Female	Male	Female	Male	Female
All causes	21,293	11,606	18,730	10,788	25,677	12,977
Infectious and parasitic diseases	308	88	231	68	370	78
All neoplasms	3,252	1,488	3,391	1,531	3,543	1,610
Circulatory disease	11,796	8,037	10,781	7,543	13,930	8,857
Pneumonia	279	118	167	80	383	101
Other respiratory diseases	1,531	523	1,228	407	1,429	381
Alcohol-related disease	455	123	201	59	863	230
Accidents and violence*	2,519	597	1,623	456	3,768	873

* Excluding accidental poisoning by alcohol.

Source: Leon *et al.* (1997).

Causes of death that are alcohol-related, as well as accidents and violence, show particularly marked fluctuations; death rates from homicide were two to three times higher in 1994 than in 1987.

However, the picture is not so clear when we consider the cause of cardiovascular disease. In the West, it is generally the case that alcohol consumption is associated with lower rates of heart disease, at least consumption that is regular and in moderate amounts. So why did a *reduction* in alcohol consumption lead to improvements in life expectancy? Why is alcohol consumption not protecting those in settings such as Russia? The answer may lie in the pattern of consumption – rather than drinking moderate amounts at regular intervals. It is the Russian cultural norm to drink large amounts in one session, known as 'binge drinking' (see also Box 4.13). Russians are also much more likely to consume liquor such as vodka, rather than wine or beer. When vodka has been home-brewed, its alcoholic strength is unknown, and it can be very potent and therefore very dangerous. Patterns of consumption such as this are more likely to produce rather than to prevent health problems.

There is thus some persuasive evidence that drinking habits may be responsible for much of the high mortality rates observed in the region in the early 1990s. However, if such 'behavioural' factors do underlie many health outcomes, these behaviours themselves need to be put into context – we need to ask the questions such as 'why do people drink in this way?'

Social and socio-economic factors – consequences of the transition from communism

Drinking culture in what is now the former Soviet Union is something that needs to be seen in the context of both cultural norms and the role of the state.

Box 4.13 Binge drinking among young people

Binge drinking is commonplace among young people, especially college and university students, in countries such as Australia, Britain and the United States. It is often an integral part of college culture and a mainstay of socializing. Those who are involved in fraternities or sororities and also sports clubs are particularly likely to be binge drinkers. Binge drinking is defined as five or more drinks in a row for men and four or more drinks in a row for women, with a standard bottle of beer, glass of wine or shot of liquor each counting as one 'drink'. Binge drinking can lead to blood-poisoning, and also to accidents, violence and even suffocation in one's own vomit.

The deaths of a number of students as a result of binge drinking have led to many campus educational campaigns and attempts to change the social norms surrounding binge drinking.

As in many countries, the consumption of alcohol has long been a central aspect of socializing, and drinking large amounts, even to the point of collapse, was considered the norm. This was for many years supported by the position of the centralized Soviet state, which saw alcohol as the one 'consumer' good that it could easily supply to the population. Apart from brief periods such as Gorbachev's anti-alcohol campaign, alcohol was cheaply and readily available. Cultural demand and state supply were thus mutually reinforcing.

However, alcohol has not only cultural and social aspects, but also a psychological facet. Many people facing personal crises, whether material or emotional, find solace in alcohol. The massive socio-economic changes that brought an end to the Soviet system had a very real impact on the lives of millions of people. The end of communism in central and eastern Europe brought new freedoms and opportunities, but it also introduced unemployment, greater inequality, and uncertainty. Death rates rose most for those with low education, the unemployed, the widowed and divorced.

The cities within Russia that experienced the highest rise in death rates, Moscow and St Petersburg, were those that also had the highest rates of labour turnover, higher average earnings but also greater unemployment and income inequality and high crime rates. This change in material circumstances and structures and the accompanying social dislocation left many people feeling disappointed and disoriented, perhaps producing a form of post-communist anomie (see Chapter 2). Watson (1995) noted an incongruity between aspirations and the means of achieving them in her study of mortality patterns in eastern Europe. The 1950s had been a period of rapid economic growth. In the 1960s, however, the increasing wealth and consumerism of the West became ever more visible, yet the socialist economies lost their dynamism and were not able to meet these western-style aspirations. These frustrations accumulated and were compounded in the early 1990s, when economic freedom and consumerism were for most people so near and yet so far – for example, consumer goods became available in the shops, but few people could afford to purchase them. In addition to this while life under the Soviet system was very restrictive, it was also very certain, yet people now had to face job insecurity, unemployment and economic instability. Thus political and economic changes on the societal level provide the backdrop for changes to people's everyday living circumstances, and ultimately can affect their health outcomes.

Section summary

Through this brief review of the unprecedented falls in life expectancy observed in parts of central and eastern Europe in the first part of the 1990s, we can see that a range of factors, or independent variables, are likely to play a part, but we cannot pinpoint any single cause. Instead, with issues such as this, we have to unpick events carefully, study trends closely and look at the detail of patterns, in this case, for example, focusing on causes of death, age-groups and time trends, in order to work out the relative importance of independent variables and how they are interrelated. Factors such as patterns of alcohol consumption, which on one level might be considered issues of lifestyle choice or individual behaviour, are integrally connected with the broader material circumstances of society.

From the regional to the local

So far in this chapter we have considered the health of countries as a whole, and just as other uses of averages hide variation, so does this. Within countries there can be great geographical and social variations in life chances, and we explore some examples of those here. First we look at variations at the regional scale, and then we focus at the smaller, local scale.

Regional variations in health

The boundaries of countries are often determined by war and colonization. Because national laws and norms are usually common across a country there are often good reasons for international studies being conducted at this level (other than the problems of obtaining data at smaller levels). However, within countries there are also great variations to be found in the patterns to people's lives – most notably between richer and poorer regions of the country. Regions are difficult to define and different countries choose to subdivide their territories in different ways for different purposes. Whatever divisions are used, however, they usually reveal variations in health which can help us further to understand how health is influenced by the nature of society as it varies over space.

Rather than comparing different countries, which can mean comparing very different population sizes (does it really make sense to compare Luxembourg to Russia?), if we use regions as our geographical unit then we are making a much more sensible comparison in terms of population. As units they are still large enough to be robust in a statistical sense and allow us to look at relatively rare causes of death or short periods of time. However, problems of data comparability mean that studies which include the regions of different countries are not commonly conducted.

Mackenbach and Looman (1994) conducted a study that looked at living standards and mortality across the regions of the European Community, using data from the 1980s. (Note that at the time of this study the 'European Community' included: Belgium, Denmark, France, West Germany, Greece, Ireland, Italy, Luxembourg, Netherlands, Portugal, Spain and the United Kingdom.) These researchers were intrigued by the fact that while at the individual level living standards are related to health outcomes, at the national level within the European Community this relationship was not apparent. Might this relationship be confounded by other variables (see Box 4.14)? Perhaps looking at the regional level could shed some light on this issue?

Mackenbach and Looman looked at regional variations in mortality using all-age standardized mortality ratios as the health outcome. The indicators of living standards that they looked at were largely driven by the availability of data, and were: GDP per capita, car access (indicating disposable income) and unemployment (indicating economic hardship). The analyses they performed were all weighted by the population size of the regions (see Box 4.15). Three potential confounders were also considered: population density, agricultural employment and industrial employment.

The results indicate that the highest mortality rates (in the 1980s) were to be found in Ireland and the northern parts of the United Kingdom, a northern Portuguese region, southern Belgium and Luxembourg, and West Berlin. The living standards in most of these regions were below the European Community average: GDP and car access relatively low, unemployment relatively high. Many of the regions with the lowest mortality also had unfavourable living conditions and the relationship between mortality and living standards was on the whole weak. However, these associations are *confounded*. After controlling for the three confounding variables there is a stronger relationship between living standards and mortality, with unemployment being the most potent factor.

Box 4.14 Confounding

We say that the apparent association between two variables, the independent variable A and the dependent variable B, is *confounded* when there is a third variable, C, which is actually causing the variation in B. For example, if we are trying to explain why the babies of some young mothers are more likely to die we might look at the mothers' rates of smoking. However, these rates may simply reflect their general levels of poverty as we know poorer women are more likely to smoke.

This third variable (in this case poverty) is called a *confounding* variable.

We often need to *adjust for*, or *control for*, confounding variables in order to be sure of a relationship between our study variables.

Box 4.15 Weighting

When comparing areas or groups of different sizes, it often makes sense to weight the analyses by the size of those groups. If this is not done then the significance of the relationship between the study variables in a relatively small population, such as Luxembourg, will have as much 'weight' or influence as the significance of the relationship between the study variables in a relatively large population, such as Germany.

It seems that the effects of urbanization and industrialization on increasing premature mortality had obscured the mortality-lowering effects of high living standards.

Britain experiences some of the highest rates of ill health in Europe in some of its regions, but health in the south of the country is among the best in Europe – so we now turn to this divide. It is often the case that health divides within countries are greater than those between them.

Britain: the north–south divide

Britain has long been scarred by geographical inequalities in health. Differences in mortality rates between rural and urban areas have been reported, with the latter usually experiencing higher rates. Recent research shows that spatial inequalities in mortality continue to persist today. Table 4.6 shows age-standardized mortality rates for both men and women. Substantial geographical variations in mortality are apparent, both between countries of the UK and between regions of England. At the regional level within England, there is evidence of a clear north–south divide. For deaths at all ages, the northeast and northwest have the highest mortality, and the southeast, southwest and east of England have the lowest mortality rates. This regional inequality is less marked, however, for deaths occurring at younger ages.

Other research has focused at a smaller geographical scale, using old county borough boundaries so that changes in mortality from the 1950s to the late 1990s can be seen (Mitchell *et al.*, 2000). This spatial categorization divides Britain into 292 areas. This work also uses a different technique for looking at geographical patterns in mortality over time. At each time period for which data were available, Britain was divided into ten equalized groups of areas in terms of population – these are called deciles. The standardized mortality ratio (SMR) of each of these groups was then calculated. Table 4.7 shows starkly that spatial inequalities in mortality in Britain have been polarizing since the early 1980s. In 1990–92 people living in the decile area with the highest mortality rates were 42 per cent more likely to die prematurely than the national average; this rose to 50 per cent higher in the period 1996–98 and to 53 per cent in 1999. The types of areas that make up decile 1 are predominantly in the north, whereas those on decile 10 are mainly in the south.

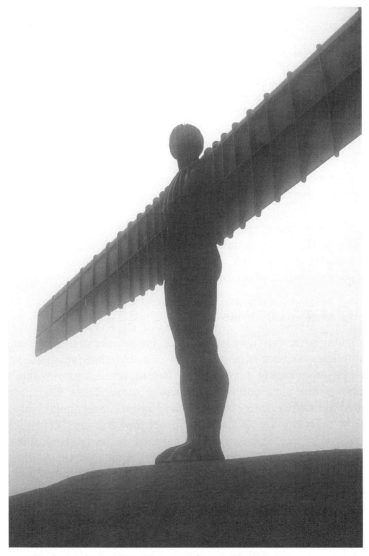

Figure 4.10 The Angel of the North, near Gateshead, England.

Source: Photograph by Mary Shaw.

Unemployment and health

Traditionally, one of the most significant factors studied at the regional level is unemployment. Unemployment is often treated as solely a socio-economic category pertaining to an individual, but it is also clearly a very spatial variable. An individual cannot find work, no matter how qualified and experienced they may be, if there are no jobs available within reasonable distance of where they live.

Table 4.6 Age-standardized mortality rates for all causes of death by country and government office region (GOR), 1991–97 (rates per 100,000)

	Men					Women				
	All ages*	1–14	15–44	45–64*	65 and over†	All ages*	1–14	15–44	45–64*	65 and over†
United Kingdom	980	23	113	810	6,500	620	17	60	490	4,200
Great Britain	980	22	112	800	6,500	620	17	60	490	4,200
England & Wales	960‡	22	109‡	780‡	6,400‡	610‡	17	59‡	480‡	4,200‡
England	960§	22	109‡	780‡	6,400‡	610‡	17	59‡	470‡	4,100‡
Northeast	1,100§	24	108‡	950§	7,300§	700§	18	58	580§	4,700§
Northwest	1,060§	25§	124§	920§	7,000§	680§	18	66§	550§	4,600§
Yorks and the Humber	1,000§	25§	105‡	820§	6,600§	640§	20§	60	500	4,300§
East Midlands	950§	22	103‡	750§	6,400	620‡	17	59	480‡	4,200‡
West Midlands	1,000§	23	105‡	810	6,700§	630§	17	60	490	4,300§
East	870‡	20‡	93‡	650‡	6,000‡	570‡	16	53‡	420‡	3,900‡
London	970‡	22	129§	830§	6,300§	600‡	17	61	480‡	4,000‡
Southeast	870‡	19‡	97‡	670‡	5,900§	570‡	14‡	54‡	410‡	3,900§
Southwest	870§	20	103‡	670‡	5,800§	550§	16	56‡	420‡	3,800§
Wales	1,000§	24	117§	830§	6,600§	630§	17	63	510§	4,300§
Scotland	1,140§	25	144§	1,050§	7,300§	730§	19§	74§	620§	4,900§
Northern Ireland	1,070§	26§	125§	870§	7,100§	660§	20	59	520§	4,500§
Country inequality¶	1.19	1.16	1.33	1.35	1.14	1.20	1.19	1.25	1.32	1.20
Region inequality¶	1.26	1.31	1.38	1.46	1.26	1.27	1.38	1.24	1.41	1.24

* Rounded to the nearest 10.
† Rounded to the nearest 100.
§ 95% confidence interval excludes and is higher than the UK rate.
‡ 95% confidence interval excludes and is lower than the UK rate.
¶ Ratio between the rate in the country of the UK or the region of England with the highest rate and that with the lowest rate.

Source: Fitzpatrick and Kelleher (2000).

Table 4.7 Age–sex SMR for deaths under 65 in Britain by deciles of population (grouped by old county borough and ranked by SMR), 1950–99

Decile	1950–53	1959–63	1969–73	1981–85	1986–89	1990–92	1993–95	1996–98	1999
1	131	136	131	135	139	142	147	150	153
2	118	123	116	119	121	121	121	122	124
3	112	117	112	114	114	111	113	114	114
4	107	111	108	110	107	105	107	108	109
5	103	105	103	102	102	99	99	99	100
6	99	97	97	96	96	94	95	96	95
7	93	91	92	92	92	91	92	93	92
8	89	88	89	89	89	87	87	88	85
9	86	83	87	84	83	80	80	80	81
10	82	77	83	79	78	76	75	75	74
Ratio 10:1	1.60	1.75	1.58	1.70	1.78	1.87	1.98	2.01	2.08

Sources: Mitchell *et al.* (2000), Shaw *et al.* (2001).

Conversely, in times (or areas) of low unemployment, jobs will be relatively easy to come by, whatever the individual characteristics of the workers.

Research has shown that unemployment has a detrimental affect upon a person's health. Those who are unemployed have, in the main, low incomes, and this will have a direct effect upon living standards and eventually health outcomes. However, it seems that unemployment also has an *independent* effect on health in addition to the material difficulties it presents. There is evidence that people who experienced unemployment for more than a short period of time have an increased risk of adverse health outcomes. Morris and colleagues (1994) studied more than 6,000 men aged 40–59 over a five-year period, comparing those who had experienced some unemployment over that time with those who had retired and those who were continuously employed. They found that compared with those who had been in continuous employment, those who had been unemployed at some point over the five-year study period were almost twice as likely to die in any year. This effect was found when factors such as social class and health-related behaviours (smoking, alcohol consumption and body weight) and also health status at the beginning of the five years had been taken into account. Those who experienced unemployment were thus not more likely to die just because they smoked more, nor because they were more likely to have been previously employed in an unskilled job or because they were ill at the start of the five-year period. Instead, it appears that unemployment *per se* has a detrimental effect upon health.

Here again we can see that economic circumstances can have social and psychological repercussions. Unemployment can not only bring financial hardship, but it can also lead to social isolation and to loss of self-esteem. The context of work may sometimes provide physical hazards and emotional stress for some people, but there are also many potential benefits: self-respect, gaining the respect of others, physical and mental activity, the use and development of skills, interpersonal contact and social status. It is not surprising then that unemployment can often lead to depression and anxiety and lower levels of psychological well-being, and in extreme cases can lead to hopelessness and suicide.

Social class: diseases of affluence and poverty

We noted in the first section of this chapter that mortality trends in western industrialized nations which have passed through the epidemiological transition are dominated by chronic diseases such as heart disease and cancer, and that these are termed 'diseases of affluence'. However, this is a misnomer, as within these countries, it is not the affluent but the relatively poor who are more likely to be afflicted with these diseases. Just as the poor were more likely to suffer from cholera and plague in previous times, so they are now more likely to die younger from cancer or from a heart attack.

Despite the fact that socio-economic health inequalities in general seem to be ubiquitous in western nations, knowing to what extent and how these inequalities vary in different places might provide us with a more comprehensive picture of the nature of these inequalities and how they can be reduced. The work of Kunst and colleagues (1998) has found that mortality was higher in men working in manual occupations than in those working in non-manual occupations in all of the western European countries they studied (see Table 4.8).

When looking more closely at differences in the mortality of men aged 45–59, comparing manual and non-manual groups according to groups of cause of death, it is consistently found that the death rates of manual groups are higher than those of non-manual groups. The size of that difference is very

Table 4.8 Mortality rate ratio (95 per cent confidence interval) comparing manual classes with non-manual classes for major groups of causes of death in men aged 45–59, 1980–89

Country	All causes	Neoplasms (cancers)	Cardiovascular diseases*	All other diseases	External causes†
Finland	1.53 (1.49–1.56)	1.39 (1.32–1.47)	1.48 (1.42–1.53)	1.60 (1.48–1.70)	1.76 (1.66–1.87)
Sweden	1.41 (1.38–1.44)	1.18 (1.13–1.23)	1.36 (1.31–1.40)	1.83 (1.72–1.93)	1.76 (1.65–1.87)
Norway	1.34 (1.30–1.39)	1.25 (1.18–1.33)	1.34 (1.27–1.40)	1.51 (1.40–2.16)	1.42 (1.29–1.54)
Denmark	1.33 (1.30–1.36)	1.21 (1.16–1.26)	1.28 (1.23–1.33)	1.62 (1.54–1.70)	1.36 (1.27–1.45)
England & Wales	1.44 (1.33–1.56)	1.21 (1.05–1.39)	1.52 (1.36–1.71)	1.74 (1.40–2.16)	1.74 (1.24–2.46)
Ireland	1.38 (1.30–1.46)	1.39 (1.24–1.55)	1.27 (1.17–1.38)	1.66 (1.43–1.93)	1.66 (1.33–2.07)
France‡	1.71 (1.66–1.77)	1.71 (1.61–1.82)	1.35 (1.26–1.45)	2.09 (1.97–2.22)	1.72 (1.57–1.88)
Switzerland	1.35 (1.29–1.39)	1.44 (1.35–1.54)	1.08 (1.01–1.15)	1.75 (1.60–1.91)	1.39 (1.26–1.53)
Italy	1.35 (1.28–1.42)	1.43 (1.31–1.55)	1.17 (1.07–1.28)	1.60 (1.43–1.80)	1.22 (1.03–1.46)
Spain	1.37 (1.34–1.39)	1.33 (1.29–1.38)	1.19 (1.15–1.22)	1.52 (1.46–1.57)	1.80 (1.68–1.93)
Portugal	1.36 (1.31–1.40)	1.21 (1.05–1.21)	1.03 (0.97–1.10)	1.65 (1.55–1.76)	2.15 (1.94–2.38)

* Cardiovascular diseases include ischaemic heart disease ICD 410–414, cerebrovascular disease ICD 430–438 and other cardiovascular diseases ICD 390–459.
† External causes are ICD 800–999 and include accidents, suicide and homicide.
‡ Confidence intervals for specific causes of death are estimates.

Source: Kunst *et al.* (1998).

similar in most countries, although it is somewhat greater in Finland and notably higher in France. The pattern also varies by groups of causes of death between countries. There is little occupational difference in death rates for neoplasms (cancers) in Sweden, Norway, Denmark, England and Wales, and Portugal, for cardiovascular diseases in Switzerland and the Mediterranean countries, and for external causes in Norway, Denmark, Switzerland and Italy. The class inequalities in health of the nineteenth century that were apparent when looking at infectious diseases are thus still clear today with non-infectious diseases.

Figures 4.11 and 4.12 show differences in life expectancy in England and Wales from the early 1970s to the late 1990s, for men and women respectively. We can see that life expectancy for all classes has risen, but also that class dif-

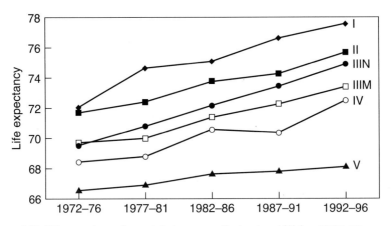

Figure 4.11 Life expectancy by social class, men, England and Wales, 1972–96.
Source: From data in Hattersley (1999).

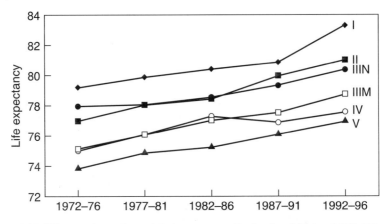

Figure 4.12 Life expectancy by social class, women, England and Wales, 1972–96.
Source: From data in Hattersley (1999).

ferences in mortality have persisted, and that for men especially, they have widened in the most recent period.

Section summary

As should be apparent from the studies we have referred to above, a person's location in terms of their country and region has an influence on their health, as does their social location and the times they are living through. Studies often include one or two of these dimensions but rarely all of them. Next we take a more detailed geographical view. By looking at the very local level we can begin to see the interplay of all these influences.

Local variations

In this last section of the chapter we consider studies of health at a much smaller geographical scale. By 'local' we refer here to studies that look at an area such as a town or city. These are sometimes general studies about the state of health in an area, or they can have a very specific focus, such as investigating a particular outbreak of disease. The focus, of course, will depend upon the research question at hand.

At this local, or neighbourhood, scale there has been a great deal of research on the relationships between 'types of neighbourhood' and the 'types of people' who tend to live in them. While bigger areas such as counties or states tend to have, on average, a wide variety of people living within them, neighbourhoods often contain quite specific groups of people at similar stages in their lives, with very similar economic or family circumstances, similar racial identities and similar attitudes to the world. The processes that operate to bring these patterns about are called 'residential differentiation' and have been widely researched and written about by urban geographers and sociologists such as Harvey (1989) and Soja (1980). These processes are driven by a combination of economic (such as the housing market) and social processes (such as identification with a particular group of people and a desire to be part of that group).

This body of work is relevant to us because it reports that very extreme contrasts in the nature of the population can be found within very small distances in towns and cities. Since we know that the residents' characteristics (especially their social and economic markers) will affect the levels of ill health in an area, these sharp divisions from neighbourhood to neighbourhood may well be reflected in sharp divisions in health – just a couple of streets' distance can take you from one level of ill health to another.

Here we present some examples of research on this smaller spatial scale. The first compares two cities with similar socio-economic profiles but very different mortality rates (Middlesbrough and Sunderland, UK), the second refers to a town which at one time enjoyed particularly low mortality rates relative to neighbouring areas (Roseto, USA), and the third looks at a place where death rates are generally relatively low but there are pockets of higher mortality (Oxford, UK). Each of these examples gives an idea of the questions that can be posed and the insights that can be gained from focusing at the local level.

Example 1 Middlesbrough and Sunderland, UK (Phillimore and Morris, 1991)

This piece of research looked at two cities in the northeast of England which appeared to be equally deprived in economic and social terms – Middlesbrough and Sunderland. However, premature mortality in the early 1980s was markedly and consistently higher in Middlesbrough. This pattern was apparent for both sexes, for all age groups and for many causes of death.

The researchers looked at a number of factors that might explain this discrepancy, including the socio-economic histories of the two places in the early twentieth century, the possible role of unmeasured poverty, individual lifestyle factors, differences in the provision and use of health services and differences of the built environment and in atmospheric pollution.

They gathered and presented a wide range of data with which to compare the two areas, but their analysis stands out most for the way that they pose questions and delve beyond standard measurements. For instance, as well as looking at the economic well-being of the two areas, they consider the *dynamics* of economic indicators such as unemployment rates. They note that while unemployment has been consistently high in Sunderland, Middlesbrough has experienced periods of 'boom and bust'. They ask: 'Is it possible that the subsequent dramatic decline into widespread deprivation, rather than the absolute level of deprivation itself, is one cause of Middlesbrough's excess mortality?'

One factor they did not consider in great detail, however, was migration (see Chapter 6). Their data showed that Middlesbrough experienced a higher turnover of people – but they did not follow up this clue as to why the two cities, otherwise very similar, might have such different health outcomes.

Example 2 Roseto, Pennsylvania, USA (Wolf and Bruhn, 1993)

In the 1970s US researchers noticed that the small town of Roseto, home to approximately 1,600 people, had had relatively low death rates, and that this had been the case since the 1930s. The death rates for heart disease were particularly low. However, this could not be explained by the usual risk factors for heart disease: diet, smoking and exercise.

Wolf and Bruhn conducted a study of the town to try to understand the reason for these low death rates. After looking beyond the usual statistical factors, they found that the town was largely made up of descendants of Italian-American immigrants who had arrived in the 1880s from the town of Roseto in Italy. It was noted that they formed a particularly close-knit community, where family and civic ties were strong, and far more potent than in other towns in Pennsylvania. Wolf and Bruhn saw this community as characterized by strong social cohesion with a clear egalitarian ethos – people supported each other rather than competing with each other. The researchers thought that these social conditions explained the relative health advantages enjoyed by Roseto residents.

However, Wolf and Bruhn noted that from the 1960s these community ties began to loosen, and the younger generation began to move away from the town. The town became more affluent and materialistic values became more prominent. As the researchers predicted, as the sense of community and the ethos of egalitarian values waned, the health advantage was also lost. Again, note the reference to migration in this study.

Example 3 Oxford, UK (Brimblecombe *et al.*, 1999)

This study explored the relationship between housing tenure and health. Using standardized mortality ratios for deaths under 65 (SMR < 65) as an indicator of health, the city of Oxford as a whole had a mortality rate which is very close to the national average. In the period of this study (1981–92) the SMR < 65 for Oxford was 96, just 4 per cent below that for England and Wales. However, calculating SMR < 65 for electoral wards within Oxford, which each contain on average 7,000 residents, reveals that at this more local level the SMR < 65 range from 65 in 'North' ward to 130 in 'South' ward. Those living in 'South' ward are thus twice as likely to die before reaching the age of 65 than those living just a few miles away in 'North' ward.

Although at the national level there is a clear relationship between housing tenure and health outcomes, at this local level there is no significant relationship between tenure and SMR < 65. The explanation for this lies in the composition of tenures of individual wards and in a much more qualitative consideration of tenure. For example, interviews with key informants (local people working in the housing sector) revealed that owner occupation varies tremendously from one part of the city to another in terms of the quality, value and condition of houses, the facilities of the area and the economic and social situation of those who live there. Privately rented accommodation varies too, from very high-quality accommodation to extremely poor quality, unsafe and unhealthy accommodation.

Likewise, there was no significant relationship at the ward level between deprivation (using the Townsend score) and mortality, despite there being a well-established relationship on a national level. However, mortality was related to the proportion of the population who were unemployed, and to the proportion on income support. These measures may be more sensitive (in this context) to people's actual living standards – than a measure of their tenure. Those living in privately rented accommodation, for example, could be on relatively high incomes or they could be unemployed and claiming benefits. While housing tenure can generally indicate social position, at this local level it can be misleading, especially when the cost of renting can vary considerably even within a small locality.

A closer investigation of housing and housing tenure in Oxford revealed that the ward with the highest SMR < 65, 'South' ward, also had the highest proportion of homeless people and there were three hostels for the homeless in the ward. Thirty-nine out of the 161 male deaths in 'South' ward over the study period were among those living in hostels for the homeless, or living in hostels at some point in the last six months before their death. Recalculating the SMR < 65 for 'South' ward excluding these 39 deaths meant that the mortality rate for the ward became 107 – much closer to the national and Oxford average.

A relatively small group of people, in this case homeless people, who have a particularly high risk of dying young, can thus affect the mortality rate of a small area, which otherwise contains a fairly affluent, and healthy, population. Yet again, migration had a part to play (the homeless group were all migrants, either from other areas of the city or from elsewhere in Britain).

Conclusion

Through this chapter we have looked at a number of spatial scales and how patterns of health can vary from the global to the local. We have also looked at how health can vary along a number of sociological dimensions, by social class, gender and age. And we have seen how other social processes, such as large-scale structural social change, and health behaviours in their social and cultural context, affect the health of people of different social groups and people in different places. We have also used a number of different measures of health, and defined some key methodological concepts. Here we have focused on variations between places and between groups of people and some possible explanations for the patterns observed. In Chapter 5 we look more closely at disentangling those social and spatial patterns and the extent to which differences between areas are due to composition or context. In Chapter 6 we turn to the role of social and spatial migration in creating and maintaining health inequalities.

It is worth thinking at this stage about how you can keep all these intervening factors in your mind at once – let alone how researchers can include them all in their studies. One way of doing this is to think about a small area at a particular point in time and to ask yourself how the health of the residents of that place may be influenced by living there, then, by who they are and what they do. If you ever find the discussion here becoming too complicated think 'how did I fit into the areas in which I have lived and how do I interact with society – in which ways might this affect my health?'

Further reading

- There are a number of atlases of disease and mortality available which are worth studying, for example:

Holland, W. (ed.) (1988) *European Community Atlas of Avoidable Death*. Oxford University Press: Oxford.

Cliff, A. and Haggett, P. (1988) *Atlas of Disease Distributions, Analytical Approaches to Epidemiological data*. Blackwell: Oxford.

Glover, J. (1999) *A Social Health Atlas of Australia*. University of Adelaide, Public Health Information Development Unit: Adelaide.

- If you found the section on central and eastern Europe interesting then you will find this book informative:
  Cockerham, W. (1999) *Health and Social Change in Russia and Eastern Europe*. Routledge: London.

- Essayist Sontag, who has herself recovered from cancer, presents her thoughts about how we view illnesses both old and new, and what that tells us about the way we view the world:
  Sontag, S. (1989) *Illness as Metaphor* and *Aids and its Metaphors* (in one volume). Doubleday: New York.

Suggested activities

- Look at the World Health Organization and UN websites and their reports. The *World Health Report* is an annual publication and is available on-line.
- Look at published statistics to find out how your country compares with others in terms of its health and other indicators.
- Search for a study of health in your local area, using the Internet or your local library.
- Search for up-to-date articles on a particular topic, such as mortality rates in central and eastern Europe, using a database such as *Medline*. How has the debate moved on since we wrote this chapter?

References

American Association for World Health (1997) *The Impact of the US Embargo on Health and Nutrition in Cuba*. American Association for World Health: Washington, DC.

Bennett, N., Bloom, D. and Ivanoz, S. (1998) Demographic implications of the Russian mortality crisis. *World Development*, 26: 1921–37.

Bhatti, N., Law, M., Morris, J., Halliday, R. and Moore-Gillon, J. (1995) Increasing incidence of tuberculosis in England and Wales: a study of the likely causes. *BMJ*, 310: 976–9.

Bobak, M. and Marmot, M. (1996) East–West mortality divide and its potential explanations: proposed research agenda. *BMJ*, 312: 421–5.

Botting, B. (1997) Mortality in childhood. In Drever, F. and Whitehead, M. (eds) *Health Inequalities*. The Stationery Office: London, pp. 83–94.

Brimblecombe, N., Dorling D. and Shaw, M. (1999) Where the poor die in a rich city: the case of Oxford. *Health and Place*, 5(4): 287–300.

Bunting, J. (1997) Appendix A: sources and methods. In Drever, F. and Whitehead, M. (eds) *Health Inequalities: Decennial Supplement*. The Stationery Office: London.

Curtis, S. and Taket, A. (1996) *Health and Societies: Changing Perspectives*. Arnold: London.

Fitzpatrick, J. and Kelleher, M. (2000) Geographic inequalities in mortality in the United Kingdom during the 1990s. *Health Statistics Quarterly*, 7: 18–31.

Harvey, D. (1989) *The Urban Experience*. Blackwell: Oxford.

Hattersley, L. (1999) Trends in life expectancy by social class – an update. *Health Statistics Quarterly*, 2: 16–24.

Kubik, A., Parkin, D., Plesko, I., Zatonski, W., Kramarova, E., Mohner, M., Friedl, H., Juhasz, L., Tzvetansky, C. and Reissigova, J. (1995) Patterns of cigarette sales and lung cancer mortality in some central and eastern European countries, 1960–1989. *Cancer*, 75: 2452–560.

Kunst, A., Groenhof, F., Mackenbach, J. and the EU Working Group on Socioeconomic Inequalities in Health (1998) Occupational class and cause specific mortality in middle aged men in 11 European countries: comparison of population based studies. *BMJ*, 316: 1636–42.

Leon, D., Chenet, L., Shkolnikov, V., Zakharov, S., Shapiro, J., Rakhmanova, G., Vassin, S. and McKee, M. (1997) Huge variation in Russian mortality rates 1984–94: artefact, alchol, or what? *The Lancet*, 350: 383–8.

Mackenbach, J. and Looman, C. (1994) Living standards and mortality in the European Community. *Journal of Epidemiology and Community Health*, 48: 140–5.

McKee, M. (2001) The health consequences of the collapse of the Soviet Union. In Leon, D. and Walt, G. (eds) *Poverty, Inequality and Health*. Oxford University Press: Oxford.

Mitchell, R., Dorling, D. and Shaw, M. (2000) *Inequalities in Life and Death: What if Britain Were More Equal?* The Policy Press: Bristol.

Morris, J.K., Cook, D.G. and Shaper, A.G. (1994) Loss of employment and mortality, *BMJ*, 308: 1135–9.

Moss, A., Hahn, J., Tulsky, J., Daley, C., Small, P. and Hopewell, P. (2000) Tuberculosis in the homeless: a prospective study. *American Journal of Respiratory and Critical Care Medicine*, 162(2): 460–4.

Office for National Statistics (ONS) (1997) *Mortality Statistics: General. Review of the Registrar General on deaths in England and Wales, 1993–1995*. Series DH1 no. 28. The Stationery Office: London.

Patel, T. (1994) *Fertility Behaviour: Population and Society in a Rajasthan Village*. Oxford University Press: Delhi.

Phillimore, P. and Morris, D. (1991) Discrepant legacies: premature mortality in two industrial towns. *Social Science and Medicine*, 33(2): 139–52.

Roberts, I. and Power, C. (1996) Does the decline in child injury mortality vary by social class? A comparison of class specific mortality in 1981 and 1991. *BMJ*, 313: 784–6.

Shaw, M., Dorling, D. and Davey Smith, G. (2001) Did things get better for labour voters: premature death rates and voting in the 1997 election. Townsend Centre for International Poverty Research, University of Bristol.

Sontag, S. (1990) *Illness as Metaphor* and *AIDS and its metaphors* (in one volume). Doubleday: New York.

Soja, E. (1980) The socio-spatial dialectic. *Annals of the Association of American Geographers*, 70(2): 207–25.

UN (2000) *Human Development Report, 1999*. UN: New York.

UN (2001) *Human Development Report, 2000*. UN: New York.

UNAIDS/WHO (2000) *AIDS Epidemic Update: December 2000*. WHO: Geneva.

Watson, P. (1995) Explaining rising mortality among men in Eastern Europe. *Social Science and Medicine*, 41(7): 923–34.

WHO (1998a) *World Health Statistics Annual 1996*. World Health Organization: Geneva.

WHO (1998b) *Burdens of Disease 1997*. World Health Organization: Geneva.

WHO (1999a) *Reduction of maternal mortality*. A joint WHO/UNFPA/UNICEF World Bank Statement. WHO: Geneva.

WHO (1999b) *Removing Obstacles to Healthy Development*. World Health Organization: Geneva.

Wilkinson, R.G. (1996) *Unhealthy Societies: The Afflictions of Inequality*. Routledge: London.

Wolf, S. and Bruhn, J. (1993) *The Power of Clan: A 25-year Prospective Study of Roseto, Pennsylvania*. Transaction Publishers: New Brunswick, NJ.

SECTION II

Chapter 5

Health inequalities: composition or context?

Chapter summary

In the previous chapters of this book we have presented a general introduction to some of the ways in which medical geographers and medical sociologists think about the world and how they carry out research. In this chapter we present a more detailed exploration of an issue that is at the centre of numerous current debates and discussions within the discipline. This is the issue of differing health outcomes among social groups and among areas, which is generally referred to as 'health inequalities'.

This issue concerns a fundamental question about the causes and distribution of ill health in western industrialized societies and has ramifications for every aspect of the discipline and for any policy implications that stem from our research. We are going to discuss this question using two key terms: *composition* and *context*. We will thus begin with a definition of those two terms, move towards an explanation of the central questions which they provoke, examine why this is such a key issue in medical geography and medical sociology and then consider aspects of the issue in more detail.

Introduction: composition and context

Where the chances of good or bad health are not evenly distributed among groups of people (defined either by the area in which they live or work or by some other common characteristic), we say that there is *health inequality*. The context/composition question is all about explaining those health inequalities. If people in an area are markedly more unhealthy compared with people in another area this might be because the population in the worse off area contains a higher proportion of *individuals* who are at greater risk of ill health, or it

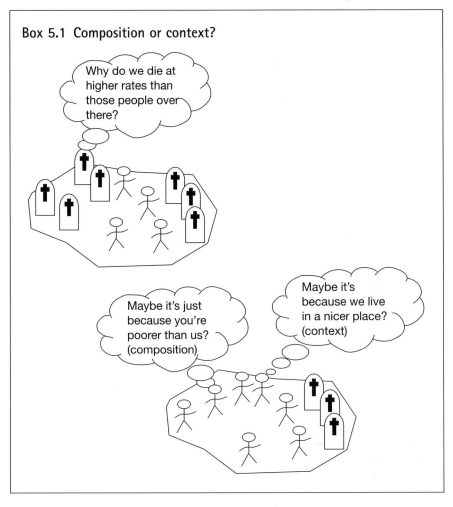

Box 5.1 Composition or context?

might be because there is some feature of the *context* in which they live – of their physical, economic or social environment – that is raising their chances of being ill. The first explanation is referred to as *composition* because it hinges on how the population is made up of different kinds of people. The second explanation is called *context* because it hinges on the setting in which people live their lives.

Box 5.1 illustrates the essence of these ideas. The essential point to grasp about these two different approaches to explaining health inequalities is that *composition* locates the understanding of inequality at the *individual* level. The population's health is seen as an *aggregate* of the health of its individual members. If the *composition* explanation is entirely correct, it is assumed that there are no effects of the environment in which a person lives over and above their individual characteristics. Thus, by knowing the characteristics of individuals, we will be able to explain differences in health among populations. An

127

explanation based on *context* puts the understanding of health inequalities beyond the individual and we would expect their environment to have some effect upon their health.

The type of factors that are considered to be individual or compositional include: age, sex, smoking and diet, and various measures of socio-economic position, such as social class, poverty or wealth. Contextual factors can be things such as the health (and other) services available in an area, whether the area is rural or urban, the presence of a factory (perhaps emitting pollution) and the absence of leisure and sports facilities. Alternatively these contextual factors may be about the less tangible features of the social context – such as sense of community and group cohesion or perhaps rates of crime and the fear that crime produces. However, it is not always the case that factors can be neatly classified as either compositional or contextual. For example, an individual can be unemployed, but we can also think of areas as having high or low unemployment. Likewise, we might think of individuals as being poor, but we may also think of areas as poor, deprived or rundown. Diet can be a product of what food is available where you live (or is customarily eaten), as much as what you choose to eat. Thinking through these issues is part of the challenge of trying to understand health inequalities.

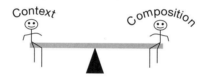

Similarly, researchers who work in this field do not believe that these two types of explanation for health inequalities are mutually exclusive, that one or the other provides a complete explanation of health inequalities. Rather, the question is one of balance. *How much* of the health differences between different groups or different areas is accounted for by population composition or by the context in which those populations live? Furthermore, other factors such as how the population moves about (considered in the next chapter) or the context within which research is carried out (considered in the final chapter of this book) can also influence how health inequalities are understood. Here, however, we are concentrating on composition or context.

In the rest of the chapter we will explore this question, drawing on some empirical evidence and thinking through the issues that the evidence raises. Before we do that, however, we feel that it is important to understand why context/composition is an important question to pose. The question comes up in many debates other than health, the most famous of these being the nature/nurture debate about human ability. To what extent are people born with potential and to what extent is their potential nurtured by the environment in which they grow up? That is too big a question for this book – we stick to tackling the context/composition question in relation to health!

Why are health inequalities important? _____

Equality

In Chapters 3 and 4 we touched on issues of equity and equality in health across the world and more specifically some of the inequalities that pervade western societies. We believe that in an ideal world, everybody should have the same chances of enjoying good health and a long life. The reality of life in western societies is a very long way from that ideal. Enormous health inequalities persist among different countries, different parts of the same country, or even different parts of the same city – as was shown in Chapter 4. We have also seen that there are differences in health outcomes between richer and poorer folk, between men and women, and between those with opportunity-filled lives and those with far fewer opportunities. These health inequalities are of considerable concern for governments, for those planning a country's health service and, we would argue, for anyone with a social conscience. At the basis of any attempt to tackle these health inequalities there must be a model that explains how these inequalities arise and how they are maintained. If we do not understand how health inequalities are created and maintained, we cannot make effective policies to redress them. Here we begin the process of constructing such a model; we then elaborate on this in subsequent chapters.

Policy implications

The tension between a compositional and contextual explanation of how health inequalities arise and are maintained also creates a debate between viewing health inequalities as a problem to be tackled at an individual level as opposed to a problem that should be tackled at a broader area level. Consider the different policy implications from your own perspective. Suppose for a moment that you have very little money, live in an extremely deprived neighbourhood, are unemployed, approaching late middle age and have begun to experience declining health. Suppose the government has two policy propositions: (1) to change the tax/benefit system so that you have more money in your pocket, or (2) to direct extra resources into the community facilities (including the health service) in your neighbourhood (see Box 5.2). Which would you choose? Why?

Research that considers the role of context and composition in relation to health inequalities has been gathered at very many different geographical scales and using a variety of sociological concepts, looking at very many different health outcomes, at different age and sex groups, and using a vast range of statistical techniques. In the rest of this chapter we do not attempt to present a systematic review of these findings but instead draw on a few examples of research that have contributed to the debate. Remember, this is a book about how to think as a medical geographer or medical sociologist might do and therefore we will concentrate on the concepts rather than the detail. If you are interested in more detail or more examples, read the relevant academic journals (see Box 5.3).

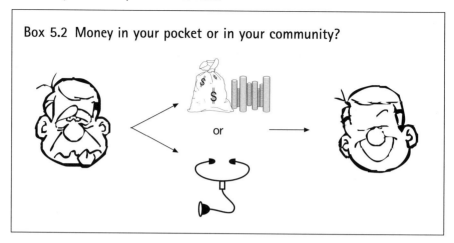

Box 5.2 Money in your pocket or in your community?

Box 5.3 Sources of information on the context/composition debate

Journals to look out for

Articles that address issues of health inequalities, as well as social and spatial aspects of health more generally, can be found in the following academic journals:

American Journal of Epidemiology	*Health Statistics Quarterly*
American Journal of Public Health	*International Journal of Epidemiology*
BMJ (British Medical Journal)	*Journal of Epidemiology and Community Health*
Critical Public Health	*Journal of Health and Social Behaviour*
Epidemiology	*Journal of Public Health Medicine*
Environment and Planning A	*The Lancet*
European Journal of Public Health	*Public Health*
Health	*Social Science and Medicine*
Health and Place	*Sociology of Health and Illness*
Health and Social Care in the Community	

Evidence

As the term 'debate' implies, there is evidence that both composition and context contribute to producing health inequalities, although what that contribution is may vary for different groups of people, in different places and over time. To get started we are going to take four examples of research that each explore this issue at a variety of scales but all in one country: Britain. These examples will introduce a number of the key techniques and concepts that surround and fuel the composition/context debate.

Boxes 5.4 to 5.7 contain just a few examples of the range of literature that describes research exploring the balance between context and composition as influences on health. They show that evidence is available to suggest that both compositional and contextual factors play key roles in determining health inequalities and that the balance between them might be different for different health outcomes, for different areas or for different groups or people. Thus it does not seem implausible that individuals might differ in their susceptibility to contextual influences on their health, or that the strength of contextual influence might vary from group to group or area to area. Such variation in the balance between context and composition is a fine example of the difficulty in trying to develop a general theory of how health inequalities are brought about, based on empirical research which can only ever have a restricted view of the world. It also makes trying to understand *how* context might influence health even more difficult.

Box 5.4 Example 1: What if Britain were more equal? (Mitchell *et al.*, 2000a)

What is the research about?
This research (already mentioned in Chapter 3 and referred to again at the end of Chapter 7) sought to map and explain changes in the geographical pattern of mortality in Britain between the early 1980s and the early 1990s.

Why is this relevant?
The research used census data to take a composition-based look at the geography of health inequalities in Britain and to ask how much of the pattern of mortality and the change in that pattern can be understood using four basic population measures. The implication is that the amount of variation in mortality across Britain which cannot be explained using composition might be explained through context.

How was the research carried out?
This research used basic techniques (see Chapter 3). It extended the calculation of SMRs (standardized mortality ratios, see Box 3.21) for deaths under the age of 65 for parliamentary constituencies across Britain, taking into account not just the age and sex distribution of the population but also the social class and employment status of the populations.

What were the results?
This research found that in 95 per cent of parliamentary constituencies, an understanding of four compositional factors – age, sex, social class and employment status – explained nearly all of the *change* in mortality rates between the early 1980s and the early 1990s. However, there were specific areas of the country for which these compositional factors did not explain (or 'account for') the change in the pattern of mortality.

What can we conclude from this?
(1) That the balance between composition and context, in terms of which is more important in determining patterns of mortality, might be different in different parts of the country. (2) That in many areas of Britain the composition of the population is more important than the context in which they live when accounting for patterns of premature mortality.

▶

Box 5.4 (continued)

But?

This research took a relatively crude approach, working at large spatial scales and with relatively few characteristics with which to describe a population. In particular the research did not explore whether additional compositional variables would have explained the patterns of mortality in those areas where unexplained patterns remained. Nor did it consider the role of migration.

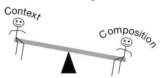

This research suggests that composition has a stronger influence on geographical inequalities in health than does context. The political implications are that macro-scale socio-economic policy (which determines wealth and unemployment rates across the country) is extremely important in creating, increasing or reducing health inequalities.

Box 5.5 Example 2: Do attitude and area influence health? (Mitchell *et al.*, 2000b)

What is the research about?

This work was about trying to *measure* the context of an area in a manner that might be directly related to health, while trying to include the possibility that the influence of an area might be different for different types of people. The work looked at the whole of Britain.

Why is it relevant?

The research used individual survey data to ask questions directly about the balance between individual characteristics (composition) and area characteristics (context). In particular, it focused on the issue of how context might actually influence health, and tried to statistically separate the size of the influence on health drawn from individual characteristics and area characteristics.

How was the research carried out?

This work employed a technique called multilevel modelling (see Chapter 3, Box 3.26). The research tried to consider which characteristics of areas might influence the health of the residential population by looking at the variable of industrial decline experienced between the early 1980s and the early 1990s.

What were the results?

The research showed that area context (measured by industrial decline) did indeed have an impact on the risk of poor health over and above the influence of individual characteristics (in this case age, sex, social class, employment status and attitude to life in the community). Individuals who had the same characteristics, but lived in areas with different industrial histories, have different risks of ill health. The size of the contextual influence was, however, relatively small. A variable which captured 'attitude to the community' (intended to be a marker of involvement in the community and thus exposure to its context) was also related to the risk of ill health. People who held a positive attitude to their community appeared to experience a lower risk of ill health.

Box 5.5 (continued)

What can we conclude from this?

This research shows that context can have a statistically significant influence on the risk of ill health for a resident population. It also demonstrates that an individual's attitude to their neighbourhood or residential area may also have an effect on their risk of ill health. However, the research suggests that compositional influences are far stronger than contextual ones.

But?

This research used multilevel modelling, which imposes restrictions on the ways in which research questions must be asked. Perhaps, most significantly, multilevel modelling demands precise specification of the area from which the contextual influence on an individual's health is assumed to originate. This can result in a mismatch between our understanding of how people perceive and use their neighbourhoods and the way in which we are trying to model that (this is akin to the difference between 'space' and 'place' touched on in Chapter 3, Box 3.10).

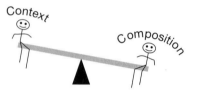

This research suggests that composition has a stronger influence on geographical inequalities in health than does context, although it did find firm evidence for some influence of contextual effects. From a policy perspective it suggests that both macro-scale socio-economic policy and micro-scale schemes to ensure vibrant, communicative, friendly neighbourhoods would both contribute to reducing health inequalities.

Box 5.6 Example 3: Social and local variation in the use of neighbourhoods (Macintyre and Ellaway, 1998)

What is the research about?

This research stands in contrast to the first two examples because its focus is at a very much smaller spatial scale. The research looked at four contrasting areas within Glasgow, Scotland, and used survey data to explore the relationships between characteristics of the neighbourhood, characteristics of the individuals in the survey sample and their propensity to undertake 'health-promoting activities'. The research directly tested the influence of neighbourhood context on individual health behaviour.

How was the research carried out?

This research was based on data drawn from lengthy face-to-face interviews. The data gathered included information about health behaviours, including the ability to socialize, take exercise and buy food locally. Information about the individuals'

Box 5.6 (continued)

socio-economic status was also obtained. A simple analysis followed whereby the odds ratio (see Chapter 3) for each of these health-promoting activities was calculated having controlled for the individuals' sex, age and social class.

What were the results?

The research showed differences between the four neighbourhoods in terms of the health behaviours of the surveyed residents. Even after taking account of the residents' individual characteristics considerable differences in the behaviour of residents from the four different neighbourhoods were found. In fact, surprisingly, once the type of neighbourhood was taken into account in the statistical model, social class was no longer related to health-promoting activity (as we would expect it to be).

What can we conclude from this?

In this case it would appear that neighbourhood context has a stronger influence than neighbourhood composition on the nature of health-related behaviour amongst the surveyed Glasgow residents.

But?

One interesting aspect of this research is that it was carried out in an area of Britain which the research in Example 1 (Box 5.4) identified as perhaps somewhere that contextual influences are unusually strong. The research is based on a relatively small sample, though the results are statistically robust. The research also differs from the other examples in that it is focused on health-related behaviours rather than on actual health outcomes.

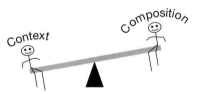

This research suggests that context has a stronger influence on geographical inequalities in health than composition. Policymakers in the health and welfare fields might achieve success by taking note of differential access to and uptake of potentially health-promoting activities in different sorts of areas.

Box 5.7 Example 4: Problematizing gender (Emslie *et al.*, 1999)

What is the research about?

This research was mainly focused on gender differences in health but includes an interesting viewpoint from which to explore how context and composition influence the health of a group of bank employees.

Box 5.7 (continued)

How was the research carried out?

The researchers undertook a postal survey of employees of a large British bank. The survey gathered both individual characteristics and perceptions of the working environment from which measurements of work context could be derived. Health outcome was measured in terms of the number of physical symptoms reported. Statistical analyses explore the relationships between context, composition and health.

What were the results?

The research showed that individual characteristics (sex, socio-demographic factors and occupational grade) were *not* related to reporting higher numbers of physical symptoms (composition) but when the measurement of perceived working conditions was included in the analysis, significant relationships with health outcomes were demonstrated. The perceived context of work (in terms of lack of job stimulation, job drain – how physically and mentally tiring an occupation is – and physical conditions at work) was the key determinant of an adverse physical health outcome.

What can we conclude from this?

In this case it would appear that context has a stronger influence than composition on the health outcome. This research stands in contrast to the other examples cited because in this instance the context is not geographical area of residence but the social context of work.

But?

The researchers also examined the relationship between composition, context and symptoms of psychological malaise. With this particular health outcome the balance between composition and context was slightly different, with individual characteristics (notably sex) having a stronger role to play. This suggests that the balance between context and composition may be different for different health outcomes.

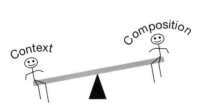

This research suggests that the influence of context is stronger than that of composition but that this balance may vary according to the health outcome explored.

Mechanisms

One aspect missing from these brief examples is any detail on *how* context might actually influence health, over and above individual characteristics. It is perhaps intuitively easier to grasp that a collection of people who are at a higher *risk* of ill-health or death might have higher rates of illness or death (for example, if they like to drive their cars very fast) than it is to conceive that some

Box 5.8 Think about where you live today

1 Imagine that you are 10 years old – do you think that playing in your neighbourhood is safe and healthy? Why? Why not? Are there neighbourhoods you know of that would be better or worse to play in? What makes them that way?

2 Now you are back at your real age. Do you think that life in your neighbourhood is safe and healthy? Why? Why not?

3 Now you are 75-years-old and living alone. Do still think that your neighbourhood is a safe, healthy place to live in or do you think that it could be contributing to the likelihood of you meeting your maker very soon? Why? Why not?

4 If you are currently in good health, imagine you have contracted a debilitating disease that means that you cannot drive and have had to give up work. Now do you think that your neighbourhood would make any difference to your health? In what way? If you are not in good health at the moment do you think that your neighbourhood has played any part in making you ill, or prevented you from getting better?

5 If you could change five things about your neighbourhood that you think would improve your chances of good health and those of your neighbours, what would they be?

6 If you could change five of your neighbours which ones would you change and why?

7 If somebody gave you a street map of your area and asked you to draw a line showing the boundaries of your neighbourhood, could you do it and where would you draw those boundaries?

8 How much time do you spend within those boundaries? How easy is it for you to escape them?

9 Think about your next-door neighbour. (Do you know them?) Do you think that they would give different answers to the last two questions?

10 Why do you live where you do? To what extent is your location (context) determined by your own individual characteristics (composition)?

feature of their residential location might affect their chance of ill-health or death (such as the design of the road system). The next part of the chapter focuses on this key question: 'How could context influence health?' To assist you in beginning to think about *context* answer the questions presented in Box 5.8. They require some thought about your own circumstances.

The questions in Box 5.8 raise a number of issues. The contrast between questions 1, 2 and 3 illustrate how day-to-day life and its relationship with health differs for people of different ages. For a 10 year old, the relationship between neighbourhood and school may be extremely important – determining activities and associates. In early and mid-adult life it is more likely that the neighbourhood which provides a place of residence is only one part of life; there may also be important work and leisure environments. In retirement and old age the neighbourhood may again become the dominant theatre in which life is lived. As activity and vulnerability change through the lifecourse, so interactions with and influences drawn from the neighbourhood may alter.

Question 4 specifically raises the different relationship between a healthy individual and their neighbourhood and an unhealthy individual and their neighbourhood – the way in which 'neighbourhood' assists or impedes life for those living with illness is an important factor to consider here. The environment where you live might not make you ill, but it might prevent you recovering quickly, or at all.

Did your answers to question 5 contain changes to the nature of the social environment (such as having friendlier neighbours) and to the physical environment (such as reducing pollution or clearing rubbish)? Which of the changes you suggested do you think would be easiest to implement? Which would be most beneficial for your own (and your neighbours') health? Did your answers include trying to change the way in which your neighbours behave towards each other?

Question 6 focuses attention on how the quality of your neighbours influences the quality of your life. Neighbourhoods differ enormously in how well residents get on together, how they interact and support each other and in the nature of the 'community' they create. What health benefits do *you* bring to your neighbourhood? Do the five people you have opted to remove from your neighbourhood damage your health? Do you believe that neighbours can influence anyone's health?

Questions 7, 8 and 9 allude to some of the more technical questions about how we research the relationship between context, composition and health. One particular difficulty that medical geographers and medical sociologists face is how to draw boundaries around the areas and how to classify the groups of people they wish to study. We have to impose these definitions on places and people, assigning people as residents of a 'town' or as members of a certain social class, for example, but these may differ from people's own views of their social and spatial affiliations, if indeed they have any. The problem is that the boundary of those areas or groups may well be slightly different for each member of the group or resident in the area. The statistical tests we use demand precisely defined areas or group membership, but we know that this is not how the 'real world' works. Researchers are therefore put in a position of having to make a hard definition of neighbourhood or group boundaries when in fact no such hard definition exists for the population being studied.

Question 10 focuses your attention on the processes that govern and constrain an individual's choice of residential location. Constraints on residential location are a key mechanism by which the people living in a particular area tend to be similar in many ways. These constraints are discussed in more detail in Chapter 6 – but basically a group of residents with similar characteristics often come to be living in the same place because of the context of that place. Most obviously they could all afford to live there but most could not afford to live somewhere 'nicer'. In turn living in that place might affect their health, but we could ascribe their health to them having similar individual characteristics when in fact they just happened to have similar individual characteristics because of the context! Trying to disentangle cause from effect is never simple.

Let's now take a more structured approach to thinking through how context might influence the health of individuals. We will make a distinction between context drawn from the physical environment and that from the social environment.

Physical/environmental context

An obvious example of how the physical environment can influence the health of individuals is the case of pollution (we have already referred to the case of pollution from power stations in central Europe in Chapter 4). Here we present some rather more extreme examples to illustrate this point. Box 5.9 gives some basic information on radiation and Box 5.10 and the map in Figure 5.1 present information about the Chernobyl disaster – a major explosion at a nuclear power station in Ukraine which occurred in 1986.

There are a some particularly interesting features of the Chernobyl example which are relevant here. The first is the inability of science to be absolutely certain (in a statistical sense) of the health impact of events surrounding the explosion at the power station. A second is the fact that although we might expect the greatest health impacts from Chernobyl to have resulted from the physical exposure to radiation, research in the region is suggesting that the psychological impact of living through the disaster, and of living with its consequences, has perhaps been as damaging as exposure to the radiation itself.

Box 5.9 The health effects of radiation

How can radiation cause harm?
Ionizing radiation literally breaks apart atoms and molecules, causing many types of damage to living organisms, depending on the type of radiation, the target organ, and the intensity and duration of the exposure. Radiation can promote or cause cancer because it damages DNA in cells. DNA is the set of instructions telling that cell what to do, how to grow and when to stop growing.

How much exposure is safe?
The answer to this depends on who you ask! In general, the regulatory approach is to try to reduce exposure to artificial ionizing radiation to zero, save for medical exposure.

Good and bad?
There is little doubt that very large doses of radiation are bad for you, but remember that different kinds of radiation are useful and benefit your health. X-rays, for example, are only possible because of the way your body responds to radiation.

Source: Radiation Reassessed at http://whyfiles.org

Box 5.10 The Chernobyl nuclear power station disaster

- On 26 April 1986 the Chernobyl nuclear power station in Ukraine suffered a major accident which was followed by a prolonged release of radioactive substances.

- Fallout was detected not only in northern and in southern Europe, but also as far away as Canada, Japan and the United States. Only the Southern Hemisphere remained free of contamination.

- Acute health effects occurred among the plant personnel and those who participated in the emergency phase to fight fires, provide medical aid and help with the immediate clean-up operations. A total of 31 people died as a direct consequence of the accident, and about 140 suffered various degrees of radiation sickness and health impairment. No members of the general public suffered these kinds of effects.

- In the decade following the accident there has been a real and significant increase of cancers of the thyroid among the children living in the contaminated regions of the former Soviet Union, which could be attributed to the accident.

- An important effect of the accident is the appearance of a widespread state of psychological stress in the affected populations. This phenomenon appears to reflect public fears about the unknowns of radiation and its effects, as well as the public's mistrust towards public authorities and official experts. It is certainly made worse by the disruption of the social networks and traditional ways of life provoked by the accident and its long-term consequences.

- Radioactive contamination from the accident cannot be blamed for *all* the illnesses reported. Other factors must be considered:
  - Much of the affected population had never previously received what we would consider to be modern, adequate health care. The extensive medical surveillance of these people after the accident may be uncovering medical problems and conditions that already existed but were not apparent.
  - There are many gaps in the medical data for this region for the period before the accident in 1986, especially concerning specific illnesses and causes of death. As a result, it is difficult to measure the health impact of the Chernobyl accident because there are often no baseline data with which to compare the post-accident statistics.
  - The latency period, i.e. the time it takes for cancer to develop, for solid cancers (cancers other than leukaemia and thyroid cancer) is usually at least 10 years. In spite of lurid reports of thousands of new cancer cases since the accident, it can be argued that there has not been sufficient time to determine the extent of Chernobyl-related cancers.

For more information see: http://www.uilondon.org/uiabs95/bebabst.htm

The case of Chernobyl shows how important the collection of routine health statistics can be. Without reliable information, regularly collected, we cannot make sound judgements as to the effect of specific incidents such as this. Even if a great deal of health information is collected after an incident, unless there are comparable measures from before that incident we cannot be sure of the

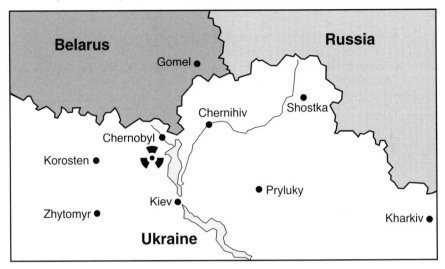

Figure 5.1 The location of the Chernobyl nuclear power station, Ukraine.

effect of the radiation. This example also shows how studying the influence of a factor of the physical environment can be problematic. In the case of Chernobyl, the original site of the explosion can be easily located in a geo-

---

Box 5.11 Coal workers' pneumoconiosis (black lung)

- Black lung occurs among coal miners. It is a work-related disease caused by continued exposure to excessive amounts of coal dust. The dust becomes embedded in the lungs, making breathing very difficult.
- The symptoms of black lung include shortness of breath, coughing and painful breathing. Black lung may result in permanent disability and premature death.
- The Federal Black Lung Program in the United States provides just under $460 million annually in monetary and medical benefits to former coal mineworkers disabled by pneumoconiosis.
- Between 1931 and 1948 over 22,000 British miners were forced to leave their work because they had pneumoconiosis – 85 per cent of these workers lived in South Wales.
- Smoking does not increase the prevalence of pneumoconiosis, but, because it can damage lung function, it may exacerbate the symptoms of the disease.
- In 1999 the UK government agreed the largest ever industrial injury compensation pay-out. Around £1.5 billion will be paid in damages to 65,000 former miners suffering from debilitating lung diseases. The miners took legal action against the government and the nationalized coal industry, claiming it had been known for decades that dust produced in the coal-mining process could cause lung disease and that not enough had been done to protect them.

For more information on 'black lung' see: www.webmd.lycos.com

graphical sense, but the geography of the radioactive fallout is far less precise. Moreover, the psychological impacts of the explosion are even less tangible but may have affected a far greater number of people. The migration of people away from the affected area is also a factor to take into consideration. People may move away from the contaminated area as a consequence of the disaster, and from a research point of view this migration might affect findings concerning the health effects of the disaster (see Chapter 6 for a fuller discussion of mobility, migration and health). Consider now another environmental context – coal mining (Box 5.11).

In our second example we consider how a feature of the physical environment affects not a group of people in a particular geographical area but those working in a particular profession. Box 5.11 gives a few details of 'black lung', a disease encountered by those continually exposed to coal dust or dust containing a high level of silica. Legal battles both in the United States and in Britain were fought throughout the 1960s, 1970s, 1980s and 1990s in order to gain compensation for those workers whose health was damaged by unavoidable exposure to harmful substances through their work. Much of this legal wrangling centred on proving a relationship between work, exposure to dust and subsequent disease. In Britain the legal battle mirrored this chapter's discussion of the balance between composition and context in many ways. One legal argument suggested that the individual characteristics (the health-related behaviour and social class) of the mineworkers were the true cause of illness among that occupational group. The other suggested the context of their work was the root of their illness. This is a stark indication of the relevance of these kinds of academic discussion to the real world.

Box 5.12 and Figure 5.2 provide our third and final example of a physical environment contextual influence on health. The natural presence of radon gas and its collection in buildings presents a health hazard both in parts of Britain and across the United States. Radon is a gas that occurs naturally, leaking from

---

Box 5.12 Radon gas

- In parts of Britain and a great deal of the United States pollution from radon gas in domestic homes is a matter of concern.
- Radon comes from the natural (radioactive) breakdown of uranium in soil, rock and water and gets into the air.
- Radon is estimated to cause many thousands of deaths each year because long-term exposure to it can cause lung cancer.
- The US Congress has set a long-term goal that indoor radon levels be no more than outdoor levels, but currently indoor levels are more than three times outdoor levels.
- The US Environmental Protection Agency website carries lots more information about radon: www.epa.gov
- For the UK, www.bre.co.uk/radon is a good source of information.

Proportion of homes with long-term, living area
radon concentrations over 4 pCi/l*

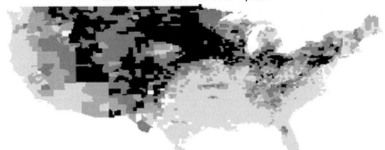

Proportion of households
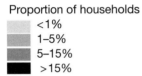
<1%
1–5%
5–15%
>15%

*In the United States, radon is measured in 'pico-Curies per litre', abbreviated pCi/l. Most homes have living-area concentrations between 0.5 and 1.5 pCi/l, but some homes are much higher. The US Environmental Protection Agency suggests that everyone in the country should test their home for radon, and that people with living-area concentrations over 4 pCi/l should take some action.

Figure 5.2 Radon in US homes.

Source: data from E.O. Lawrence Berkeley National Laboratory High-radon Project.

earth and rock and through ground water. Radon is radioactive and it is this property that means its presence and build-up in buildings can be problematic. Since people generally spend most of a typical 24 hour day at home, the levels of the gas there are of key concern. There is no question that in sufficient quantities, breathing in radon gas can cause lung cancer but there is some disagreement about what constitutes a 'sufficient quantity'. It does appear to be the case that smokers, who are already at much higher risk of lung cancer anyway, significantly exacerbate that risk by breathing in radon gas.

In the United States, many people have their homes tested to see if the radon gas levels there are 'dangerous' and maps showing those areas most likely to be at risk of radon penetration are widely available. The good news is that comparatively small changes to a home can dramatically reduce the radon levels within it. Radon levels seem to be a good example of an environmental influence on health which varies from area to area.

With these three examples we have moved from one specific incident (Chernobyl) to how the context of work can affect an entire occupational group (coal miners), to an environmental context that may affect the health of millions of people, albeit slightly. Thus context can range from the particular to the general. Environmental contexts are some of the most easy to explain and understand. The effects of social context are more difficult to pin down – particularly

142

the precise mechanisms whereby someone's poor social context can damage their health. We keep looking for evidence of these mechanisms because of the geographical concentration of people with poor health living in poor social environments. If there are indeed contextual effects on health from living in areas of poverty they are likely to be far greater than are environmental influences, but as Boxes 5.4 to 5.7 showed, finding the evidence is not easy. We now turn to the social context and the search for the mechanisms that might lead to its possible influence on health.

Social context

It is the influence on health from the social world which particularly intrigues medical sociologists. We saw in Chapter 2 that the work of Durkheim, first published at the end of the nineteenth century, explored the role of social integration and social cohesion in affecting suicide rates. This essential question of medical sociology – how the social environment is related to health – continues to elicit a great deal of interest and is the topic of lively debate for those interested in the interactions and mechanisms of health, place and society. The discussion of the role of social capital (discussed below) on the health of communities is one of the contemporary expressions of this debate.

The report in Box 5.13 is a good illustration of the relationship between health, medicine and society in which medical geographers and medical sociologists are often interested. The initiatives described illustrate an increasing trend to try to break down the barriers between clinical medicine (which takes place when an individual comes into contact with clinical doctors and the health-care system) and social medicine (which takes place in society to try to prevent or minimize the amount of contact that people have with clinical doctors and the health-care system). As societies increasingly struggle to pay for their health-care systems, interest in how society and clinical medicine are related and how they can be better integrated grows rapidly. However, as we have illustrated above, how aspects of day-to-day life in a community might influence the health of people in addition to their individual characteristics can be difficult to conceptualize and to research. We will structure our look at this topic under four headings: tangible fabric, state fabric, social fabric and equality.

Tangible fabric

By tangible fabric we refer to physical and material features of the community's day-to-day life including the nature of the housing in which people live, the shops that support them and the facilities that are available for them to use and enjoy. There is a lot of evidence to suggest that living in poor-quality housing (which is, for example, damp, cold and cramped) damages health both in a physical sense, through exposure to increased physical hardship, and in a psychological sense, through demoralization. Many researchers

---

Box 5.13 From the American News Service, by William Bole

In what appears to be a growing trend, hospitals around the country are performing radical surgery not just on their patients, but on their communities as well. Consider these recent developments:

- In Washington, D.C., a local hospital system has taken over and refurbished apartment houses owned by absentee landlords, triggering a wave of housing development and renovation in the city's poorest neighbourhoods.
- In Detroit, hospitals are supporting an effort to plant community gardens in formerly vacant lots and teach inner-city youngsters how to grow vegetables and sell them to local markets.
- In Pueblo, Colorado, hospitals have launched a 'family strengthening' campaign that involves visits by nurses into the homes of mothers considered at risk of abusing their children or themselves with drugs.

None of this would seem to be exactly what the doctor ordered. But more and more, hospitals are looking to improve the health of locals by improving the quality of community life, according to health officials and others involved in the efforts.

"A lot of things that have nothing to do with medical care nonetheless have a direct impact on health and wellness. And that's why the hospitals are reaching out," said Tyler Norris, an independent consultant who helps hospitals set up community action programs. "Decent housing providing a sanitary environment for children, neighbourhood gardens yielding fresh produce and nutritious meals, home visits helping keep young mothers and children out of the hospital – these are but a few of the initiatives that have come out of the Healthy Communities movement."

Source: Village Life, 14 April 1997.

---

also believe that the quality and price of food supplies available in the immediate neighbourhood have an impact on health and health-related behaviour. People who are not mobile are forced to shop within their immediate environment and therefore they may have a limited choice about what they buy and the amount that they pay for food. Likewise, the ability to exercise, relax and enjoy yourself (a vital component of staying healthy) is to some extent controlled by the availability and quality of facilities in the area. Most people know that taking exercise is important for their health but if the streets are dangerous (or perceived to be) and there is no park or sports centre in the vicinity then people are likely to be deterred from taking exercise. It therefore seems entirely plausible that the quality of the tangible fabric available to a community could influence the health and health-related behaviour of community members.

It is important to realize here that there is a context to what is considered 'poor' in any one time and place. What we would consider poor housing today, for instance, would have been seen as very fine housing a century ago. One of the most intriguing aspects of studying medical sociology and medical geography is that as living standards in the western world have risen, there has not been a commensurate decrease in health inequalities. The gap between the life expectancy of rich and poor has often widened for instance. Thus it may not be simply the absolute level of people's material circumstances (what they have) that influences health as much as their relative positions. People also generally live longer nowadays so that even slight environmental influences on health (such as mildly damp housing) have longer to influence their health.

Housing is just one part of the tangible social environment that can influence health: there may be direct physical consequences – unsafe electrical wiring causing fires – but there are myriad related psychological factors as well. Living in a tower block is not necessarily a bad thing – if you have a safe entrance, a working lift, plenty of space and a well-maintained apartment. But if the lift is not working, the corridors are covered with offensive graffiti and littered with the discarded needles of drug-users, and you do not feel safe even when inside your home, then your physical and mental health are likely to be affected by your housing situation (see Box 5.14 for more on the health implications of poor housing).

State fabric

 In Britain and the United States the systems of access to state support, social and medical services are organized differently (see Box 5.15). But in both settings the support and services that you receive can vary according to your own material wealth. Although the quality of medical care and basic state support services may not vary markedly across these countries, access to them and the pressure those services are under does vary markedly according to the nature of the communities they serve (again, community may be defined either spatially or socially). For example, suppose as an elderly person you require help in your home – if you happen to live in an area where the home help services are under particular pressure the quality and quantity of care you receive may differ from those in an area where the services are under less pressure.

In Britain it is estimated that the net effect of the welfare state reduces 'real' inequalities in wealth and hence the extent of inequalities in health (Shaw et al., 1999). Although there are variations across Britain in the ability of the welfare state to perform, in no part of Britain is the situation, in terms of welfare, as uneven as across many parts of the United States. This is despite the fact that the United States spends far more on health care as a percentage of GDP than does Britain. In the United States individual states decide how equitably they wish their health care and other welfare services to be spread. The state governments have a very strong role to play in determining the contexts within which people live their lives. Of course, in these two democracies people have a very strong role to play in determining the government that influences this context.

Box 5.14 The health implications of poor housing

Problems	Health implications
Outside the home	
Design and layout	Poor design and layout of housing may lead to increased stress and depression among residents, prompting violent behaviour and contributing to longer-term mental health problems. Poor design and layout may also inhibit child development.
Air quality, pollution and neighbouring houses	Outdoor air pollution and noise from neighbouring houses affects quality of life and may cause anxiety, stress and depression. Specific pollutants that are harmful to health may be passed into local ecosystems via industrial processes or accidents. Contaminated land can endanger health through the escape of contaminants into the soil.
Security	A secure environment gives comfort and confidence to residents, while poor security can lead to stress, anxiety, depression and potentially violent behaviour. There is also the possibility of physical harm to residents from intruders in the home or from street violence outside.
High-rise housing	The design and layout, and the associated quality of service provision, can have an impact on a variety of conditions including stress, anxiety, depression, violent behaviour, increased blood pressure, isolation, inhibition of child development, presence of infectious diseases and respiratory problems.
Inside the home	
Dampness and condensation	Can lead to respiratory illness, coughing, asthma, diarrhoea and gastro-enteritis, headaches and tiredness.
Poor heating and insulation	Can lead to illness and death from hypothermia, ischaemic heart disease and respiratory illness.
Poor ventilation	Increased risk of transmission of infectious disease such as TB as well as illnesses caused by damp and condensation.
Disrepair, unfitness and lack of amenities	Disrepair can make houses cold, dangerous and difficult to heat. Lack of basic amenities leads to increased rates of gastro-intestinal illness such as dysentery. Both increase levels of stress, long-term depression and anxiety.
Lead water pipes	Cause damage to the central nervous system, affect the mental development of children and cause a general reduction in the speed of reaction and reflex, possibly increasing risk of accident in the home.

▶

Box 5.14 (continued)

Inadequate noise insulation	Causes increased blood pressure and pulse rate, long-term chronic stress, headaches, depression, etc.
Structural hazards, internal layout and home safety	Increases the risk of accidents in the home: estimated to cost the NHS £300 million per annum in Britain.
Air quality	Can be affected by passive smoking, carbon monoxide, asbestos, and radon gas leading to increased risks of illness and death.
Houses in multiple occupation (buildings divided into smaller units where residents share some amenities, such as kitchen and bathroom, e.g. hostel)	Risk of death by fire increases by about 10 times. Increased risk of a range of health problems due to layout and standards increase anxiety, stress, depression, blood pressure, respiratory illness and transmission of infectious disease.
Overcrowding	Increases the risk of respiratory infection, infectious diseases such as TB and digestive tract infections such as dysentery. Lack of space increases risk from accidents and levels of stress.

Source: http://www.vois.org.uk/healthousing/html/healthimplications.htm.

Social fabric

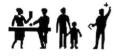

As we have already noted, the notion of community coherence and social support continues to be debated within medical sociology and medical geography. The notion that a cohesive community, in which members interact with and support each other, has better health outcomes than a socially fragmented community is not particularly new (see Chapter 2). Many researchers believe that a cohesive community is as valuable as (or may compensate for a lack of) material wealth and opportunity. A community in which people do not live in fear of crime, that recognizes and looks after those who need extra assistance, and that campaigns to improve the tangible fabric of their lives, may have real power to reduce the risk of ill health to which each of its community members is exposed. A term has emerged which is used to refer to these community characteristics which might affect the health of a community: social capital. Box 5.16 introduces some of the key issues involved.

Box 5.15 Comparing the US and UK health-care systems

The UK and US health-care systems are organized in very different ways. The UK has the National Health Service (NHS) which is funded and administered by the state, through the tax system. In principle it delivers health care to everyone, regardless of their status, for free. In practice, some (relatively inexpensive) facets of the service have to be paid for, such as prescriptions, spectacles and some dental services. Some people choose to take out private medical insurance; such schemes cover the costs of treatment beyond that which can be administered by a GP (family doctor).

The US health system is based principally on private medical insurance, with many people belonging to schemes supplied through their employment. The state does provide a basic service through Medicare (which covers those aged 65 and over or those with specific medical conditions which means that they cannot get insurance elsewhere) and Medicaid (which is available to those who are younger, but on low incomes or without adequate insurance to cover the care they need).

In practice, about 25 per cent of the US population are covered by one or other of these schemes, but it has been estimated that half the total health-care costs of the United States are met by state funding because those covered tend to be the poorer and sicker groups in the population.

Both the UK and US systems of health care share common features – unequal quality of care and waiting times throughout the population (principally between richer and poorer groups and places) and an almost constant political desire to reorganize them with the aim of saving money and/or enhancing the care they provide.

In the UK, the NHS is regarded as a sacrosanct institution. Its wholesale abolition or privatization would be political suicide for any government. However, the pressures to restrain costs (and hence the tax burden on the public) are high, often leading to intense politicization of any decisions that affect the way the NHS is run. UK governments like to be seen to increase spending on the NHS. In the United States, George W. Bush (now President) said 'I'm absolutely opposed to a national health care plan' (17 October 2000). Al Gore was in favour of moving 'step by step' towards it (18 August 2000). Both pledged to spend more to help the 'uninsured' population receive the care they need.

There are extremely strong connections between the social capital thesis and our last contextual issue, equality. Researchers are often talking about different things when they refer to social capital. At one extreme are people (such as us) who believe that social capital can only be maximized when people are more equal. At the other extreme are those researchers who believe that social capital can be high in a hierarchical society where everyone knows their place and function – and is happy with their lot. It is not impossible for both scenarios to be true, but one problem with using terms that are ill-defined is that quandaries such as this can arise. Such confusion can also help account for the popularity of the idea of social capital as it is easy for many people to agree about something if it is so vaguely defined and they can impose their own interpretation!

Box 5.16 A quick guide to social capital

- Although the term social capital means different things to different theorists in different eras, in today's literature there is broad agreement that social capital is related to social interaction, membership of social networks and the consequences of these. The origins of social capital can be attributed to various authors from Bourdieu in 1986, to as far back as Durkheim (1897) or even Marx (1848).

- The idea of social capital is that through socializing, social interaction and participation in social networks, people can access a stock of resources that makes the quality of their day-to-day lives better. This pool of resources does not refer directly to money, but might include support that equates to a financial advantage. For example, a group of families who help each other with child care gain an advantage in not paying for it; they might also gain peace of mind.

- There are some specific pathways through which a stock of social capital might improve health, or at least lower the risk of illness. These include aspects of social interaction which may promote healthy behaviours (nagging from friends to visit the doctor when symptoms persist, offers of support during recuperation aiding rapid recovery, for example). They might also include the relief of stress, physical hardship and emotional difficulties through support.

- Some research has shown statistically robust associations between higher levels of social capital in communities and lower levels of ill health.

- But, social capital can be difficult to measure for analyses using a quantitative approach. Researchers disagree as to the 'best' way to measure social capital.

- An association between higher levels of social capital and better health has been seized upon by governments both in Britain and the United States as having relevance in a policy context. Governments believe if they can foster higher levels of social capital within communities, there may be tangible health benefits. This equates directly with the question which began this section – should health policy be targeted at individuals or at groups or areas? The social capital thesis suggests that work with groups or areas may be fruitful in enhancing the health of individuals. This approach stands in contrast to an individualistic one in which population health is improved by changing the behaviour and/or characteristics of individuals.

Equality

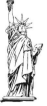

An extremely important thesis within medical geography and medical sociology contends that an equal society (in terms of material wealth and opportunity) is a healthy one. Many proponents of this thesis believe that it is *inequality itself* which leads to high levels of ill health and high mortality rates. In simple terms this means that a contextual influence on health might be the level of inequality in a community, group or in wider society. The original and most well-known proponent of this argument is Richard Wilkinson; we referred to his thesis in Chapter 4, noting that for countries beyond a certain level of national wealth the distribution of income within a country, rather than simply how rich that country is, is an important factor in determining the population's health. Here we revisit this important idea.

Wilkinson's theory acknowledges the influence of an individual's material position (their income, which is an individual characteristic), but also situates the individual within a community or an area where the degree of income equality (the context) might condition and explain the relationship between their material circumstances and their health. This theory was built upon empirical evidence that differences among affluent countries in terms of their relative level of mortality are related more closely to income inequality *within* them, than to differences in absolute income *among* them. In more simple terms, Wilkinson showed that it is not how rich a country is that explains its mortality rate relative to other countries, but rather the size of the disparity between richer and poorer folk within it. He suggested that health inequalities are primarily produced by the direct and indirect effects of 'psychosocial stresses' which are experienced differentially because of people's differing social positions. Again, in more simple terms, Wilkinson argues that it is your socio-economic position in relation to others that affects your health because of the psychological impact of being relatively poor in comparison with others. In effect, he suggests that it is simply more stressful to live in an unequal society if you are nearer the bottom of the pile, and that stress is of course strongly related to health and poor health-related behaviours.

If we consider this theory in relation to the questions posed in this chapter, the level of inequality within a community, group, neighbourhood or country can be thought of as the *context* that influences health over and above *compositional* characteristics (the material wealth of the population). Not surprisingly, this is a highly contested theory and one that is continuously reanalysed and

---

Box 5.17 A Metaphor

'First class passengers get, among other advantages such as better food and service, more space and a wider, more comfortable seat that reclines into a bed. First class passengers arrive refreshed and rested, while many in economy arrive feeling a bit rough. Under a psychosocial interpretation [following Wilkinson], these health inequalities are due to negative emotions engendered by perceptions of relative disadvantage. Under a neo-material interpretation, people in economy have worse health because they sat in a cramped space and an uncomfortable seat, and they were not able to sleep. The fact that they can see the bigger seats as they walk off the plane is not the cause of their poorer health.'

Source: Lynch et al. (2000).

---

debated as new evidence appears. Some researchers have contested it on methodological grounds, claiming that finding the effect of income inequality on average life expectancy is dependent upon which countries are included in the analysis and how income and income distribution are measured. Others have an objection which is more ideologically based, arguing that if there is an effect of income inequality on health then this is primarily due to *material* inequalities in living standards rather than as a result of pyschosocial stress (see Box 5.17 for an eloquent example of this position). Perhaps, as quantitative measures which capture elements of the social environment become more sophisticated and more widely available, better empirical evidence will be in place to help untangle this theoretical dispute.

There have been a number of attempts to connect Wilkinson's ideas on income inequality and psychosocial stress with the social capital thesis. Indeed, there is some common ground shared between Wilkinson's thoughts on the role of social cohesion (produced by low levels of income inequality) and the notion of social capital. Some argue that building social capital in communities is the way forward for reducing health inequalities, although Wilkinson is a proponent of reducing the underlying income inequalities that undermine the establishment of social capital.

Box 5.18 Take the friendly neighbour test

- How friendly are you towards your neighbours? Are you in regular contact?
- Would you/do you help them out when they need it?
- If something went wrong in your house would you first seek help from your neighbours?
- Do you invite your neighbours round for social activities?
- Do you participate in community events and/or religious meetings?
- If someone from your neighbourhood needed help would you give it readily?

Untangling context and composition

In this closing section of the chapter we further explore the relationship between context and composition. As before we will begin with some questions for you to think about.

There is almost no limit to the ways in which individual characteristics can be measured and these include descriptions and measurements of attitudes and behaviour. Answer the questions in Box 5.18.

Suppose that we have the same measure for all of your neighbours and that we find your neighbourhood consists of very supportive people who interact with each other a great deal. This information is still held in terms of individual characteristics so is this a measure of neighbourhood composition or of context?

By gathering information about individual behaviour and characteristics to a greater and greater extent, surely the potential for finding contextual influences on health becomes smaller and smaller? What is the difference between saying that an individual has access to and provides social support and saying that a neighbourhood provides social support? The neighbourhood does not exist without its constituent neighbours, but does it add up to more than the sum of its parts? If we know enough about the neighbours do we know everything about the neighbourhood context?

A second difficult set of questions to consider is the very strong relationship between some individual characteristics – and group membership or residence in particular types of neighbourhood. The relationship between 'who people are' and 'where they live' has been explored by geographers, with many concluding that the relationships between individual characteristics or behaviour and residential location are simultaneously and mutually constructive. Where you live is who you are is where you live. In that sense then, trying to make a distinction between contextual and compositional influences on health is futile and the results obtained will depend entirely on the way in which the question is asked, how the data are constructed and which of numerous possible statistical tests are performed. It is a little bit like pressing a cookie cutter onto dough and then baking the piece you cut out – the shape you get at the end depends very much on the shape of the cutter with which you began.

Indeed, many statistical techniques actually push the researcher into trying to conceptualize their questions in such a way as to suit the structure of the test. Multilevel modelling, for example, is specifically designed to measure the influence drawn from individual characteristics *and* the contextual characteristics of hierarchies of groups or areas. Given that this technique is designed to find the balance between context and composition it is no surprise that it often does so. Perhaps the relationship between individual characteristics and the characteristics of groups or areas is not well suited to analysis by quantitative techniques. In Chapter 7 we go on to show how much research is also influenced by the times and places in which it is undertaken as well as by the techniques and theories that are available at any one time and place.

We have also made much of the need to understand how health inequalities are brought about in order that they may be tackled by policy initiatives. Can this still be achieved if we begin to doubt the value of a distinction between contextual and compositional influences? We have repeatedly made reference to 'the nature of everyday life' as a source of contextual influence on health and the point at which individual characteristics and those of the group or area meet and interact. It can be argued that the best way to understand the nature of people's lives on a day-to-day basis is to talk to them about it: to use qualitative techniques. Qualitative techniques can capture and reveal far more about the relationship between individual characteristics and the nature of day-to-day lives than can quantitative techniques. Census and survey data can take a snapshot of regions or countries but may not tell us about the mechanisms that balance individual characteristics and the context of those individual lives.

Qualitative techniques can help elucidate those mechanisms for more specific areas or groups of people. Together and in balance many would argue that these two research approaches have the potential to provide the research input to policy that is required. The simple answer to the question about how or whether context and composition need to be (or can be) unravelled is that we do not yet have the answer. This is partly what makes conducting research so interesting – it is obvious that the both context and composition matter, but much less obvious just how much they matter.

Conclusion

Health inequalities between groups and areas are brought about both by differences in the composition of area or group populations and by the nature of day-to-day lives within those groups or areas. The balance detected between these influences may vary from place to place, group to group and health outcome to health outcome, but it also varies according to the research approach and techniques employed by the researcher. The researcher chooses their approach and technique based upon their skills and theoretical position – these are sometimes as strong an influence on the results obtained as the phenomena they are trying to measure and explore. There is a tension between trying to provide clear and specific answers to policymakers who want to know whether to target resources at individuals or groups/areas, and recognizing the inherent complexity of the world. We believe that individual characteristics and the nature of day-to-day lives are inseparable. What makes them so inseparable is the way in which communities are constructed. They are determinants of who moves in and who moves out of particular groups and areas. That is the subject of the next chapter. It gets more complex before it becomes more simple!

Further reading

- Annandale, E. and Hunt, K. (eds) (2000) *Gender Inequalities in Health*. Open University Press: Buckingham.
  We have made a few references to gender differences in health in this book but this is a topic deserving of far more attention, indeed a book of its own. This recent collection reflects critically upon the current status of knowledge about gender inequalities in health and develops an agenda for future research. The book covers recent theoretical and methodological developments in sociology and social policy, and the significance of changes in gender relations following wide-scale economic and social changes with respect to the mental and physical health status of men and women. The collection focuses upon gender and health within industrialized nations including Britain, North America, western and eastern Europe.
- Similarly, we have not covered issues concerning ethnicity. We recommend two sources as a good starting point:
  Nazroo, J. (1997) *The Health of Britain's Ethnic Minorities: Findings from a National Survey*. Policy Studies Institute: London.

Erens, B. and Primatesta, P. (eds) (2001) *Health Survey for England: The Health of Minority Ethnic Groups*. The Stationery Office: London.
This volume contains the most recent and most detailed epidemiological data on ethnicity and health in England.

- In order to get a real feel for the ideas of any writer you should read their original work. We highly recommend that you read the work of Richard Wilkinson:
Wilkinson, R.G. (1996) *Unhealthy Societies: The Afflictions of Inequality*. Routledge: London.
Wilkinson, R.G. (2000) *Mind the Gap: Hierarchies, Health and Human Evolution*. Weidenfeld & Nicholson: London.

Suggested activities

- Look through the journals listed in Box 5.3, either in your library or online. Try to find a recent article that relates to some of the issues discussed here, read it, then look at what work it has referenced to build up its argument. To what extent do the papers you find present arguments and evidence for compositional or contextual effects?
- Have a look at the following website: http://www.healthycities.org/. Is there a healthy city in your country? What does this organization mean by a 'healthy city'? How would you define it?
- *National Geographic* magazine – buy it, read it, look at the pictures! National Geographic is a fine means of armchair travel and should prompt you to question how the lives of the peoples it documents are affected by their own locations, cultures and characteristics.

References

Bourdieu, P. (1986) *Distinction: A Social Critique of the Judgement of Taste*. Routledge: London.
Durkheim, E. (1999, first published 1897) *Suicide: A Study in Sociology*. Routledge: London.
Emslie, C., Hunt, K. and Macintyre, S. (1999) Problematising gender, work and health: the relationship between gender, occupational grade, working conditions and minor morbidity in full-time bank employees. *Social Science and Medicine*, 48(1): 33–48.
Lynch, J., Davey Smith, G., Kaplan, G., and House, J. (2000) Income inequality and mortality: importance to health of individual income, psychosocial environment, or material conditions, *BMJ* 320: 1200–4.
Macintyre, S. and Ellaway, A. (1998) Social and local variations in the use of urban neighbourhoods: a case study in Glasgow. *Health and Place*, 4(1): 91–4.
Marx, K. (1848, 1981) *Capital: A Critique of Political Economy*. Penguin Books: Harmondsworth.
Mitchell, R., Dorling, D. and Shaw, M. (2000a) *Inequalities in Life and Death: What if Britain Were More Equal?* The Policy Press: Bristol.

Mitchell, R., Gleave, S., Bartley, M. and Wiggins, R. (2000b) Do attitude and area influence health? A multilevel approach to health inequalities. *Health and Place*, 6: 67–9.

Shaw, M., Dorling, D., Gordon, D. and Davey Smith, G. (1999) *The Widening Gap: Health Inequalities and Policy in Britain*. The Policy Press: Bristol.

Chapter 6

Health and social/spatial mobility

Chapter summary

The previous chapter worked through the debate regarding the importance of *composition* and *context* in influencing people's health. In this chapter we extend that debate by adding the importance of *movement* as an explanatory factor in determining the geography and sociology of health. The chapter explores how medical sociologists and geographers try to make sense of an incredibly complex world by using simple frameworks into which they fit observations and ideas. We begin by presenting a typology (or classification) of the different kinds of social and spatial movements which people can make in order to begin to understand the importance of mobility. We then concentrate specifically on social mobility. In this chapter we will often 'mix up' social and spatial terms. This is to try to get you thinking outside the 'boxes' or fixed ideas we are presenting. For instance, we talk about 'social immigration'.

Finding out how flexible and functional the categories of a typology are is an important means of seeing how well it works. We next discuss the effects of geographical mobility at different spatial scales before attempting to combine social and spatial mobility. We then show how, in most instances, where mobility affects health, both social *and* spatial movements are involved. After this we take an alternative view, asking how health can influence mobility as well as be influenced by it. Finally, we conclude by thinking more about frameworks, about how complex the world is, and how we cope with that complexity.

Introduction: migration, immigration and social mobility

In this chapter we start to look at issues that make the study of the geography and sociology of health more complicated and often more interesting. Many of the examples that we have discussed so far have shown how inequalities in health can be found among different groups of the population and/or among different places. However, people rarely stay still. They move, both between places and between social groups, and this movement can strengthen, change and confuse the patterns we see. We believe that the importance of mobility has been largely overlooked in studies of health to date and we hope that the ideas we present here go some way towards remedying that. Our attempt to comprehensively understand social or spatial mobility and its causes and consequences may appear very complicated, but if we disentangle the processes that we think are at play and then recombine them to produce a recognizable picture of the world – things will, we hope, become a little clearer.

The huge variations in living standards that are found across the globe (some evidence of these was shown in Chapter 4) would not have been created and could not be maintained without equally huge movements of people (and goods). Within any particular country the inequalities in health that are found are often the product of social movements (the forming of social classes and other systems of stratification, such as caste systems). These inequalities are often maintained only because of a huge degree of mobility taking place and, most often, these movements act to continually reinforce the patterns that we see today. As well as spatial and social mobility *influencing health* this chapter will illustrate how *health outcomes can themselves influence* and maintain the long-established patterns of these movements. We also consider micro-level movements here. Would this book have been written had its three authors not moved about socially and spatially as shown in Figure 1.1?

Since this chapter is about new ideas and alternative ways of viewing the geography and sociology of health, we do not give as many examples as in previous chapters – here we are arguing a case and, at the same time, trying to illustrate a way of thinking. We have no conclusive proof that what we are suggesting is right – that this *is* how the world really works – but we are using the chapter and its ideas to show you how researchers fuse new ideas, previous work and their own intuition to push research forward. We believe from some of the early results of our current research that social and spatial mobility could be a very important new area of study in terms of understanding health outcomes. This chapter shows you how we have come to believe that and how we have fitted the examples looked at in detail into a 'grand plan' of what might well be happening.

To summarize, this chapter builds on the examples shown in previous chapters which point to how social and spatial mobility may be key determinants of the geography and sociology of health. We shall begin by presenting a broad typology of the types and scales of mobility. A typology is simply a way of organizing our thoughts to try to simplify a complex picture in order to make sense of it. In our typology we differentiate between *internal* and *external* movements, between *spatial* and *social* movements and between *macro-* and *micro-*movements (see Box 6.1).

Have a look at the typology shown in Box 6.1. It provides a means of categorizing different kinds of social and spatial change. Think about the changes that have happened in your life, and to your community. Where would they fit in this typology? Even a simple typology such as this is not unproblematic. What are internal and external movements? It all depends where you draw the boundaries.

Box 6.1 Conceptual schema for Chapter 6

Spatial typology (for thinking about movements in space)	**Macro-scale examples**	**Micro-scale examples**
External – movement of people from one geographical area *into* another	Colonization of America by people from Europe, Asia, Africa and Latin America since 1492	Gentrification of the Isle of Dogs in the 1980s (a traditionally working-class district of London, which became populated by richer folk)
Internal – movement of people *within* a geographical area	Forced movement of rural Chinese to industrial cities during the revolution (within China)	A family being re-housed in a new estate, following demolition of their previous accommodation (through 'slum clearance')

Social typology (for thinking about movements in social status or circumstances)	**Macro-scale examples**	**Micro-scale examples**
External – imposition of new social structures or circumstances, on an existing population or person	The introduction of university education into a country creates a new class of people there	You win the national lottery and become a millionaire overnight
Internal – development of new social structures or circumstances from within an existing population or person	Women win the right to vote and to attend universities within a country	Impoverishment of a former coal-pit community as people become unemployed

In the following pages, particular examples of each influence are considered for movements of all types. Such a typology can very quickly become very complex, even if it starts from a simple premise. The value of dividing up the world in this way depends upon whether the typology created simplifies the world enough for you to be able to 'hold it in your head', whether other examples can be placed within it, and whether it helps you to make sense of the patterns you observe. It is only a heuristic device – an artificial construct designed to assist in the understanding of social phenomena – not a precise delineation of how societies and geographies are really organized, but it should help us move towards a greater understanding of complex issues. By starting to look across scales and both at spatial and social mobility, the typology should allow us to consider the interconnection and interaction of social and spatial processes. As this chapter will show, social and spatial processes are almost always inextricably linked.

Let's begin by thinking more about how *internal* migration affects health and vice versa. In the last century retirement migration was first seen on a large scale in the United States and Britain, often towards warmer coastal areas such as Florida and Devon. Such migration was possible partly because improving health meant that more people lived long enough to retire (health *affects* migration). Those people who migrated long distances in old age tended to live longer still (migration *affects* health). No one knows fully why retired people who migrate long distances tended to live longer. It could be that healthier people were more likely to contemplate such moves or that such migration was confounded with social status (richer people were more likely to be able to migrate greater distances upon retirement). By *internal* movement we mean that which is within pre-existing spatial and social units (recall our discussion of 'social facts' in Chapter 2). Such movement often helps to maintain the integrity of those units. A country, a city or a neighbourhood only functions because people move about within it. Many social groupings are maintained only by movement. An obvious example are families, which are created when people change their social status to become mothers and fathers, for instance. Nowadays many social class systems can only be maintained because of movement between those classes or, at least, the illusion that such movement is possible. Internal movements are thus the social and spatial changes in location that preserve current social and spatial orders.

External movements are defined here as the social and spatial movements that occur outside and between established orders. Box 6.1 gives the examples of colonization (*macro*) and gentrification (*micro*) as external *spatial* movements. The introduction of a university system to a society that previously had none (*macro*) and an individual winning a million pounds in a lottery (*micro*) were given as examples of external *social* movements. External movements may be perceived by those experiencing them as more dramatic, partly because people are socialized into interpreting these movements as threats to the social and spatial systems within which their lives are organized (see Box 6.2). Since *health* is so closely related to social and spatial orders, dramatic changes to those systems have important implications for the geography and sociology of health. Long-term changes in the geography and sociology of health tend to follow large amounts of external movement of people from one place to another or from one social system to another.

So, the typology is established. Now let's see how it can be applied to help our understanding of the social and spatial patterning of health. Although we began this book by explaining that social and spatial processes usually work hand-in-hand in creating and maintaining processes and patterns of health, we shall begin applying our typology by considering how social and spatial movements influence health *separately*. We will then bring them together. This kind of approach can often help to simplify apparently complex systems. As you will

Box 6.2 Four examples of established social and spatial orders

Nation-states/countries

Most were 'established' in the eighteenth and nineteenth centuries. Almost all now have strict border controls, an official language, a currency and welfare/tax system that discourages people from moving between them too often. New countries are still being created, although at a much slower rate than in the past. Recent examples are the reunified Germany and the countries that were formerly part of the Soviet Union. Reunification can be expected to have a great impact on the geography of health in Germany – people will mix more spatially and social systems will change. As we saw in Chapter 4, changes in the former Soviet Union have also had implications for the health of the populations there.

Cities

In the past many were walled. If you lived within the walls your life was often safer and your living standards better. Today many have 'walls' within them. These walls are usually not visible and are often demarcated by infrastructure – wide roads or railway tracks. The term 'coming from the wrong side of the tracks' comes from being perceived to have been brought up in the wrong part of a city as demarcated by railroads in the United States. One 'real' wall was the 'Cutteslow Wall' which was built to divide the affluent residents of north Oxford, UK, from a neighbouring council estate in the city of dreaming spires. A more well-known example, of course, is the Berlin Wall.

Social classes

Like nation-states the foundations of the social hierarchies we live in today were largely established in the eighteenth and nineteenth centuries. People came to be graded, respected and rewarded according to the nature of the work they did. People were divided into salaried/white-collar/non-manual and waged/blue-collar/manual jobs. Once this social order was established some movement between the groups was necessary to allow both for changes in demand for different kinds of work and, arguably, to justify the system – the chance exists to 'better yourself' by moving up the social ladder if you work hard! Alternatively, you might also slip down a rung or two if you don't work hard enough … or you are simply unlucky (despite how hard you work).

Gender

The traditional roles associated with being male and female have been changing rapidly in western societies. Nevertheless, at any one moment in time and in any particular place, cohorts of women and men are likely to behave, be rewarded and respected markedly differently. These differences in gender roles are culturally produced and are recreated through the processes of socialization – how people are brought up to think and act. For instance, some people think that men feel 'expected' to complain less about feeling poorly which might explain why they tend to visit doctors less often than women. However, when they do visit doctors they are often treated with more attention and respect (particularly by male doctors) as societies have generally presented men as being more important.

see from the following examples, it is not until the two sets of processes are combined that common everyday events are best and most easily described. Effects that are largely due to social or spatial processes working alone are few and far between (for example, the systematic privileging of or discrimination against a group because of their social position, or the introduction of an epidemic into a country through an apparently random journey). Apparently social or spatial processes are unlikely to be *purely* that (see Box 6.3). People tend not to travel at random and their propensity to travel is highly influenced by their social circumstances. Similarly, social groups are rarely distributed evenly throughout a country – they tend to be geographically concentrated (as we noted in Chapter 5). Furthermore the direction of cause is not necessarily simply from these processes to a health outcome. Good and poor health can influence individuals' and groups' social and spatial mobility too. The examples we give in Box 6.3 are for individuals but the typology can equally be applied to whole groups of people (such as a profession receiving a pay rise or an ethnic group being displaced geographically).

Each of the following three sections of this chapter is divided into subsections based on *scale*. Our first scale, *macro*, is usually large and refers to a long-term historical perspective or a global spatial context. Our second scale, *micro*, is usually local or personal, for instance encompassing class divisions within a country or the movement of people within a particular defined space. Very small-scale movements include the social arrangements of households or the micro-geography of everyday lives and their influences on health.

Just to reiterate, this is an artificial distinction. Through your lifetime your health might be influenced by a global epidemic, or your wealth (and other aspects of your life) may benefit by your migrating to an area where (partly because of the prosperity of the city to which you move) your health may benefit. Your life expectancy largely depends on the historical circumstances that have produced the general levels of health where you live. Your occupation, should you end up (or be) working, has a strong effect, as we made clear in Chapter 4. However, there are many other sources of influence, some major and others more minor.

Box 6.3 Examples of movements that are purely spatial or social

Social	Spatial
A worker is promoted to a higher-grade position within the company in which they were already working.	A family sell their 3-bedroom house and buy another similar home in a different area, but their jobs, schools and family income remain the same.
A couple buys a council house from the landlord, thereby becoming owner occupiers rather than renters, but without moving home.	A worker is transferred to another job, but at the same level, within a different branch of their firm in another part of the country.

For any individual it is possible to make the analysis of their health either very simple or extremely complex. 'They caught a cold because they had a chat with someone carrying the cold virus.' 'They died because they fell off a ladder.' These are simple descriptions of cause and effect. However, analysis at that level does not explain *why* they were chatting to that person or *why* they were up a ladder. Of course, we can continue to ask 'why' *ad infinitum*, as children often do shortly after mastering the power of speech, but that would force us all to become meta-physicists (those who aim to construct a theory of the nature of the world as a whole), which would make getting answers to policy-relevant questions rather difficult. One method we can employ in order to avoid the eternal asking of the question 'why?' is to study groups of people rather than individuals, as we advocate in this book. The origins of both sociology and geography lie in this approach, as was illustrated in Chapter 2.

However, a major problem with studying groups is that you can often end up simply *describing* a situation rather than *explaining* it (telling 'how it is', rather than 'why it is'). One advantage of considering *change* (in this case mobility or migration) is that you can observe the effect of a change in one situation, say social class, on subsequent changes in another, say health status. Since people's lives tend to change (in terms of location and/or circumstances) in different ways, those differences can shed light on the effects of one change, relative to another, helping to explain *why* we see the patterns we do. More importantly, the world itself is not static. It does not consist of a set of people who live their entire lives in the same way that they describe to an interviewer who happens to be gathering survey data at one point in time. People move and change their geographical and social positions throughout their lives and these movements can be just as important as where they started off in terms of their and their social groups' subsequent health profiles.

Social class and social mobility

In this book we are interested in the relationships between social class systems (ways in which people's lives are arranged, ordered and controlled) and their health. In this section we are interested in social class systems ranging from the global to the local, and in how they affect personal relations within the home and/or family and how they have been found to influence health. We can apply our typology to help structure our thoughts.

External social movements

Let's think at a *macro external* scale – the introduction of new social orders to whole populations will affect their health. The creation of the working class is a good example (see Thompson, 1964, and Eric Hobsbawm, 1999, for some further reading on this). Changes such as this altered ways of life for millions in just a few generations and we can think of them as *macro, external, social* movements using our typology. Systematic distinctions that are imposed on communities have large-scale impacts on people's health in both the short and long term. Consider the winners and losers in a coup d'état. Consider the French Revolution, or the Chinese, or the fall of the Berlin Wall. Overnight, people's entire way of life can alter, often with consequences for their health.

The abolition of slavery is a good example of a large-scale external change in the social order that has taken place in particular places at particular times with clear implications for health (see Box 6.4 and Figure 6.1). Slavery still exists in the world – often in the form of forced labour. This 'force' need not be social or military – it can also be economic.

There is a contentious argument that one of the precursors of the abolition of slavery in various places around the world at various times was itself health. Slavery was detrimental to the health of slaves, meaning that they were not as economically productive as they could be – because of the way they were treated they could not work as hard and did not live as long as 'free' people. The feudal systems that followed the system of slavery in many places were based on the principle that workers (serfs) had some freedoms, in that they could work for their own benefit but only after they had worked enough to satisfy their master's (landowner's) demands. Such systems were generally more stable and more productive than social orders based on slavery. The introduction of feudal systems of social organization brought with them stronger, but perhaps more complex, hierarchies. These hierarchies were reinforced, at least in the West, by institutions such as the church and the monarchy. In these hierarchies the vast majority of people occupied a place on the bottom level, existing as a class of peasant labourers. It could be argued that most people in the world still belong to this class, even if many of them no longer actually till the soil.

The next major western and then world social transition is far better documented both in numbers and in text. The creation, and in particular the success, of the capitalist social order and the power of trade brought with it unparalleled changes in society and so too in health. We will think of this change as a *macro external and social* movement, even though its global spread was often instigated through *macro external spatial* movements (colonization and trade).

Box 6.4 The general situation of African slaves

They are beaten and tortured at discretion. They are badly clothed. They are miserably fed. Their drudgery is intense and incessant, and their rest short. For scarcely are their heads reclined, scarcely have their bodies a respite from the labour of the day, or the cruel hand of the overseer, but they are summoned to renew their sorrows. In this manner they go on from year to year, in a state of the lowest degradation, without a single law to protect them, without the possibility of redress, without a hope that their situation will be changed, unless death should terminate the scene.

Source: Clarkson (1817)

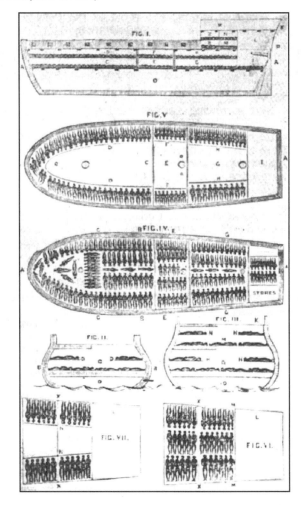

Figure 6.1 Cross-section of a typical slave ship in the eighteenth century.
Source: Howe (1972).

Capitalism is the word used to describe a form of social order that began in Europe in the sixteenth century, when the power of merchants, who had amassed wealth through trade and manufacturing, superseded the power of feudal institutions. Over the next two centuries the factory system was created (recall our description of the Industrial Revolution in Chapter 2). Economies of scale and mechanization produced more goods using fewer people, and changed the nature of labour for those who worked in the factories. Generally the *social* importance of human beings at the bottom of the hierarchy fell in relation to the *economic* importance of labour, goods and machines. The focus for most capitalists was the accumulation of wealth rather than the welfare of their workforce.

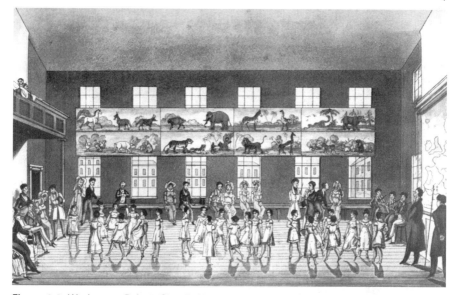

Figure 6.2 Workers at Robert Owen's New Lanark spinning mill participated in 'agreeable recreation' three times a week.

There were some exceptions, however. Robert Owen invented the notion of sickpay and health care for his labour force around this time, in New Lanark, Scotland (see Figure 6.2). The co-operative movement grew from here and unionized labour led the struggle for better conditions for workers. The study of health, place and society also began in earnest at the peak of the acceleration of this transformation, in the place that it had altered most – England – during the nineteenth century. The wealth that capitalism created allowed a group of (mostly rich) men to begin to study the health of particular people in particular places. The academic discipline of epidemiology was born out of a changing social order. Capitalism continues to control life across the world today. Individuals are alive today who have more personal wealth and power than the populations of entire countries. They are, on the whole, pretty healthy people. Figure 6.3 gives an indication of the unequal distribution of the world's wealth.

What we have tried to illustrate from the above examples is that large-scale social change might matter most in influencing the health of large numbers of people. Where there is change, there are always winners and losers. Some systems systematically favour certain groups of people and that is how inequalities in health come about. Inequalities in health and wealth, worldwide, have reached levels beyond the imagination of people only a couple of generations ago.

Internal social movement

Now let's think about *macro internal* social movement. Large-scale social change of the kind described above occurs relatively infrequently. In contrast, social

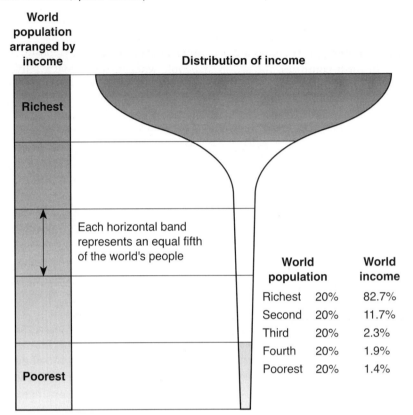

World population arranged by income

Distribution of income

Richest

Each horizontal band represents an equal fifth of the world's people

Poorest

	World population	World income
Richest	20%	82.7%
Second	20%	11.7%
Third	20%	2.3%
Fourth	20%	1.9%
Poorest	20%	1.4%

Figure 6.3 The uneven distribution of the world's wealth, 1999.

Source: British Medical Journal (1999). © BMJ Publishing Group.

migration, movement *within* a social hierarchy, is occurring all the time (although the extent of this mobility is often exaggerated). The possibility of social mobility is one part of the means by which the current social systems in which the majority of us live are justified. The ubiquitous 'American dream' (the idea that if you work hard, you can be whatever you want to be, get where you want to go) epitomizes this possibility. A few individuals live that dream and succeed in making meteoric rises up the social hierarchy. They are few enough still to be newsworthy even in an age of global media. Most people, however, stay more or less at the same position in the social scale into which they were born.

As the last two chapters have shown, your position in the social hierarchy has a great influence both directly on your health and on your health-related behaviours. The reality across much of the globe is that divisions between different social groups are widening, but that some people *do* move between those divisions. How does this movement influence health?

One common misconception is that many people move from poorer to richer social classes with the consequence that the richer social classes are becoming larger and the poorer classes are becoming smaller. In fact the opposite may be true. In most countries, the group of people who, in total, own a tenth of that country's wealth is getting smaller and smaller (and richer and richer) (the inequalities shown in Figure 6.3 are getting greater). At the same time the group who are leading more insecure lives, on relatively smaller incomes, is becoming larger. Of course, countries vary greatly according to how progressive their social policies are but very few countries have policies to counteract the growing concentration of riches. If we have seen one solid equation in this book, it is that relatively higher wealth equals relatively better health. If wealth is increasingly concentrated among a smaller group of people, improvements in health will also be concentrated there.

Part of the problem is visible if we think at a *micro* or individual level. As more people believe they have elevated themselves to a higher social status, the lines delineating social strata shift. In Britain for instance, there are many people at university who are the first child in their family to have achieved that level in the educational–social hierarchy. What is less readily appreciated is how a university degree is not quite what it used to be in terms of social value, even if its academic merit is still high (see Figure 6.4). Those with an interest in maintaining their position in the social hierarchy begin to value qualifications from particular universities only, or qualifications higher than the basic university degree. Processes of social inclusion and exclusion are thus maintained despite an apparent social change. The health implications of this are less certain. The findings of many studies suggest that higher levels of education are related to better health outcomes, but it is not clear how much of this effect is due to the

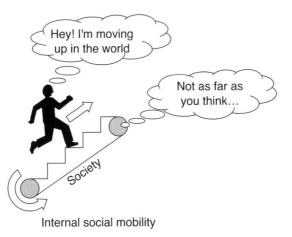

Figure 6.4 Internal social mobility.

fact that higher education leads to more occupational opportunities and thus to a higher social status and relatively better living standards. As a higher proportion of people gain higher educational qualifications, the advantage that those qualifications bring may well diminish.

For those few who do genuinely move up the social hierarchy the health gains, on average, are readily apparent. In aggregate they live much longer than their (lower-status) parents and they are less likely to suffer illness throughout their lives. The improvements in their material situation are largely responsible for this, but increasingly the sense of well-being that success brings can be seen to aid good health. In societies where social success is so highly rated it is hardly surprising that achieving higher material gain and social respect is beneficial. Increasingly, however, this is a product of what we collectively value (or what we are socialized to collectively value). Social success is also not a complete panacea. Many people believe that 'the grass is greener on the other side' but find that when they achieve success it is not necessarily what they thought it would be. Politicians often find that gaining power does not bring them the pride (and certainly not the respect!) that they thought it would, for instance. Similarly there are many tales of lottery winners discovering that the onset of untold riches does not necessarily bring them happiness. Individual self-advancement in a very unequal world is only partially beneficial. It is certainly not the mirror image of moving in the opposite direction.

For those who drop *down* the social class hierarchy, the poor health implications are striking. Moving down a social hierarchy tends to lead to loss of not only material resources, but also self-respect, friendships and often relationships. Failure scars, financially, emotionally and, ultimately, physically. One notable feature of downward social mobility is that its adverse health consequences outweigh the beneficial consequences of climbing the social hierarchy. People who are downwardly mobile suffer a greater adverse impact on their health than the benefit felt by those who are upwardly mobile (if you *did* win £1 million in the lottery then the long-term health effects would be likely to be only just noticeable; if you lost your job, there would probably be a marked negative effect). One implication of this for health at a *macro*-scale is that more socially mobile societies where lots of people are moving up and down (such as the United States or Britain), can have worse overall levels of health because the poorer health of the sizeable downwardly mobile population outweighs the health benefits gained by the upwardly mobile.

The form of social mobility most important to an individual's life and health operates at the *micro*-scale: your changing position in the hierarchies of the classroom, friendships, relationships, workplace and family. However, it can be difficult to see these processes at work among groups. If we look at the health of children in a single school year or that of a large extended family, their overall levels of health will be related to factors such as the general levels of affluence of that family or school. However, within any such group particular individuals' experiences, and their health, can vary widely. Some of that variety is often due to *micro social mobility*.

School-age children tend not to exhibit the same social gradients of ill health that their parents or younger siblings show. Social hierarchy and selection within a school or within a group of childhood friends (and adversaries) is based less on issues such as material wealth and more on individual personal skills and how children cope with major transitions such as puberty. A large, if not the largest, manifestation of ill health in school-age children, in affluent societies, is symptoms of poor mental health such as depression; eating disorders also have a high prevalence, which can be connected with self-esteem. Changes in the day-to-day, month-to-month position of children within their peer group, family and friends can have strong influences here. Becoming unpopular at school can be stressful. Health issues can be intimately related to changes in the micro social position of children – to *micro social mobility*.

In adulthood, the kind of household or family you live in, how supportive it is and how it changes over time are all of great importance to health. Friendship networks matter greatly to well-being – much research suggests that the support that they bring has a benefit for health. In much current research this often comes under the conceptual umbrella of *social capital*, which we referred to in Chapter 5. If you consider your own life – who you interact with in a typical week – and think how those experiences help or hinder you and how they make you feel, their importance should become clearer. Changes in these relationships are what we have called *micro social mobility*. Becoming unpopular at home, or at work, can be stressful. Having someone there to look after you when you are ill makes a difference. Losing the people who help care for you, or making new friends and forming new relationships, matters. At the simplest micro-level, people who are better at making and maintaining friendships are likely to live longer. Simple things, which matter for health at this *micro*-level, can be more important to you as an *individual* than your own social position or the *macro*-scale changes to society that are taking place around you.

It is important to remember here that we are still talking about averages (see Chapter 4, Box 4.6). There will always be rich people with lots of friends who are very ill, people permanently unemployed who live to 80 and the infamous 90-year-old life-long smoker. However, this does not mean that influences at the individual level are not important – it just means that we can measure their importance only by looking at groups of like individuals. As the last chapter showed, our difficulty then is in distinguishing between what is affecting the group as a whole through context, and the individual sum of the parts which represents the compositional effect on their health.

As we get old, *micro social mobility* grows even more in importance. There are many reasons for this, not least because the likelihood that you will be ill and need to be cared for grows with age. Being widowed is a major social change. Do you believe that people can literally die of a broken heart? Also, think about why the mortality curve for men 'spikes' upwards slightly at age 65. There is no biological reason for it, but in many western societies age 65 is traditionally a key time for the micro social mobility of men – they retire at this age and lose what is often their main source of social identity.

Finally, it is important to recognize that these very personal changes in people's lives are not immune from wider social changes. Within the space of a single generation it is possible to see how wider social change affects personal social mobility. A generation ago the likelihood of elderly people being cared for by their daughters was far higher than it is today. Such a role was expected of young women in the past (in particular the youngest daughter) although it may not necessarily have been explicitly stated. Today people have fewer children, and thus fewer daughters, and women have fought and partly won a battle against these ascribed social roles. It is, for instance, less likely given current trends that your children will provide care in a personal way for you, as you get older, than it is that you will provide care for your own parents.

The above discussion has looked at social mobility, at both micro- and macro-scales, and from an internal and external perspective. Now let us consider spatial mobility.

Spatial mobility

You may be surprised to find that spatial mobility and geographical position are just as important as social mobility and social position in their influence on health status. Geography can sometimes even be more important. A simple example illustrates this – if you want to predict the life expectancy of a new-born baby, what single piece of information is most useful? The answer is not sex, class, ethnicity or birthweight. The answer is the country in which they were born. Life expectancy worldwide varies by a factor of two between nation-states at the extremes (look again at Figure 4.1 showing life expectancy around the globe).

Geographical mobility matters partly because of the huge disparities in levels of wealth between *and* within countries. There is nothing intrinsic to the climate or scenery of Japan that makes it a healthier place to live than the United States. Neither country, for instance, can produce enough food to feed its own population. If someone migrates from Japan to America, however, their life expectancy will tend to move towards that of the group to which they are moving. However, for international migrants, migration itself raises a range of issues related to health. Settling in a strange country and the way in which you are treated there can have an important effect on your health. This was even more the case in the past but there has never been a time when geographical mobility did not play an important role in human life, the spread of disease and the attainment of health.

At the simplest level almost all infectious diseases only exist because of human mobility. If none of us ever left our homes most infectious diseases would be largely eradicated in a very short space of time. The more we move around and the faster and further we move, coupled with the more people we interact with while travelling, the more successfully an infectious disease can spread. The transmission of infectious diseases through geographical mobility is, however, only one (albeit clear) way in which geographical mobility influences health status.

Social mobility is just as important for the transferring of diseases. If people were truly monogamous (rather than serially) then sexual diseases could not be spread. Even if people only slept with others born in the same year as them the diseases would soon disappear. The micro social mobility of forming relationships is part of the movement required for the existence of some illnesses. Sexually transmitted diseases are amongst the easiest of examples to use to illustrate this point, but the point can be made with all forms of good and bad health – all are influenced to some extent by these changes.

Macro spatial mobility – external and internal

Large-scale, long-distance population movements can be categorized in many ways. Take a look, for example, at the *The Times Atlas of European History* (Almond, 1997). Its maps begin with the flows over centuries and decades of different groups of people into different parts of the world and end with much quicker, but often larger mass migrations. These large-scale geographical movements of populations can have a clear influence on health and we briefly consider two here: colonization and immigration.

Colonization from Europe to most of the Americas, almost all of Africa and large parts of Asia and Australia brought with it important implications in terms of health both for the populations who were colonized and for the new immigrants into these continents. For the colonized, particularly in the New World, the introduction of new diseases killed far more people than any of the violence associated with these movements. For the colonizers their health too could be damaged by moving to unfamiliar places. Westerners had few remedies for diseases such as malaria during these times. Being away from 'home' also had other more subtle effects on the health of thousands of this largely male group. The 'Home Counties' of England gained their mystical status as idyllic green rural retreats from the rose-tinted memories of the empire builders. For others, escape to the freedom to build a society they desired was of spiritual and mental benefit, even if it meant physical hardship. Later still, great wealth was amassed by some people as they exploited the natural resources they found, and exploited their fellow migrants (see Figure 6.5).

Immigration is a term we tend to use when the group of people moving into an area is less powerful than those already there. Hence it stands in contrast to colonialization, which is tantamount to a takeover of territory by a stronger group of people than the indigenous population. Often immigrants move into clearly defined areas, in which there may be a concentration of other immigrants from the same or other 'foreign' groups. This movement can give rise to clear geographical differences in health or health-related behaviours which are often noticeable and so they are explored and researched. For instance, infant mortality in the Bethnal Green area of London has been relatively low for most of the last century, despite the fact that it has always been a relatively poor area.

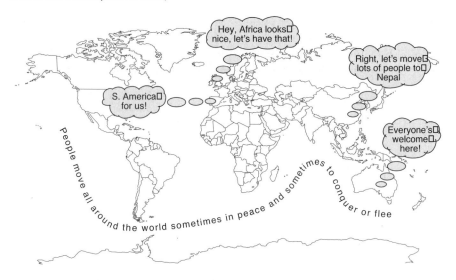

Figure 6.5 A farcical view of macro spatial mobility.

Research has associated this with the food hygiene practices of the Jewish immigrants who were concentrated there around 1900, through to the child care practices of Bangladeshi women at the end of the 1990s. However, what affected the health of these two groups *most* was that both were 'outsiders' living in areas unconsciously (sometimes consciously) reserved for 'outsiders'. Until outsiders are 'assimilated' into the general population the discrimination they suffer in everyday life, most clearly through lack of access to material resources and opportunities, is more likely to be detrimental to their health.

An extreme example of a place 'reserved' for 'outsiders' is the ghetto. The word ghetto comes from the name of the Jewish quarter of Venice. Ghettos are an extremely distinctive part of the socio-spatial map of human life and do not always form in cities, nor from immigrant populations. London for example, has no ghettos as such, despite its large immigrant population. Belfast has ghettos defined on religious grounds, formed from the indigenous populations (indigenous in terms of recent history at least). The term ghetto is most commonly associated with immigrants, however, and if you think of a city such as Los Angeles, the typical relationship between ghetto life and health becomes clear. Vast gulfs exist between health, wealth and life expectancy in the ghettos of LA, in comparison with say, Beverly Hills.

In the hierarchy of power the least powerful immigrants are termed refugees. People flee one location and arrive in another with almost nothing. Refugees are usually also the social group given the least rights and privileges when they arrive in a particular country. For instance, in Britain they qualify for the lowest levels of social security benefits in the country, are often housed in the worst housing and have to buy (or nowadays use vouchers to obtain) the cheapest food. It is hardly surprising, given their long-term and short-term circumstances, that they suffer some of the worst health outcomes.

Large-scale movement of peoples within an area or country (*internal* migration) can also affect the geography of health. When the Industrial Revolution took hold in Britain in the late eighteenth and early nineteenth centuries, people flooded from rural areas to new jobs in factories and towns. The resulting concentration of people, often on low wages and working in dangerous jobs, completely altered the geography of health. The growth of newer cities such as Phoenix in the United States illustrates that mass migration of people within a country remains practical and possible. De-industrialized communities (such as Baltimore) in the 'rust-belt' of the United States know this to their cost. Often movements of this kind contribute to the polarization of health patterns. Newer places attracting migrants tend to have better health, with the older, declining places experiencing poorer health. The evacuation of people away from Chernobyl following the nuclear accident there illustrates how events and health concerns can sometimes drive people to move internally, on a macro-scale (see Box 5.10). Initially, those that could leave did so of their own accord. Eventually, the government had to move everyone they could. Those who stayed longer would have been exposed to more radiation, therefore being exposed to greater health risks.

Figure 6.6 shows empirical evidence of the relationship between migration and health, referring to the relationship between population change in Britain over the period 1971–91 and mortality in the five years following this period. Here parliamentary constituencies are used as the geographical unit and the amount of 'population change' between the two time periods is mostly caused by migration between areas (rather than through death) – when more people leave an area than the number who enter it then the total population falls. The scatterplot shows that areas with relatively high mortality have tended to lose population, whereas those areas with relatively low mortality have tended to gain population. People have, when they have had the chance, progressively chosen to leave areas that have been poorer and where mortality is high to begin with. Similarly, people have moved into areas where life is better and where mortality was low to begin with. This is evidence of the importance of internal migration to determining and maintaining inequalities in health.

So, large-scale movements of population, perhaps over long distances, can change and shape the pattern of health in a country, city and neighbourhood. How has immigration changed the patterns of health seen in your country?

Micro spatial movement – external and internal

The grand sweeps of history and mass movements of millions of people described above may lead you to think that geographical mobility has its greatest influence at the global scale. However, there is much happening at a *micro*-scale too. Social and spatial divisions are difficult to sustain without migration. In particular, areas full of rich people need their populations to be replaced by rich

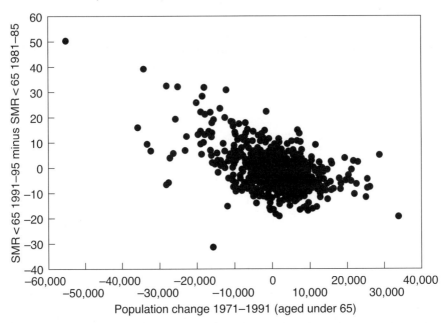

Figure 6.6 Population change (aged under 65) between 1971 and 1991 and absolute change in SMR for deaths under 65 (1991–95 minus 1981–85) for British constituencies.

Source: Davey Smith *et al.* (1998).

people and poor areas need to be filled with poor people in order for spatial inequalities to continue. The vast majority of this spatial replacement occurs through migration, and most of this occurs at the *micro*-scale. While many people pass on their home to their children when they die, it is unusual for the children then to live in that house. Instead they sell it to others, who necessarily need adequate financial resources to pay for it. In this sense, like replaces like. As an example consider London.

London has been described as the world's most cosmopolitan city. It contains more groups of people from more countries adhering to more faiths and identifying with more races than even New York (the so-called 'melting pot'). Today, partly due to immigration laws, most migrants to London come from within Britain and of those who come from outside Britain, most are from the European Union. London survives on migration. The city requires a constant influx of hundreds of thousands of young men and women in order to maintain itself. This is because it loses that same number each year as they grow older and leave the capital. London is frequently described as the conveyor belt of England. For many it is seen as a place to live in for perhaps a few years, and then move out. However, despite this vast turnover of people, from all backgrounds, races and nations, the social geography of London remains remarkably stable. Similar types of people live in the same parts of London today as they did 100 years ago. This is because the richer parts of the city have always attracted and continue to attract only those people wealthy enough to live there, and those with less money can find affordable housing only in poorer parts of the city. Again, since we know that wealth and health are related so strongly, the map of 'relative healthiness' in London looks the same today as that of 'relative wealthiness' about 100 years ago. Figure 6.7 shows a map of poverty in London in the past. This map has been compared with the map of relative poverty today and it is remarkable how little has changed (see Chapter 2).

Of course, not all of this replacement is from people coming into London from outside (external movement); it also occurs as people grow older, have families, get richer or become poorer, and so on. We can see that in this case the external/internal distinction might not be so useful in terms of distinguishing the pattern of outcomes from that movement, even if it remains useful to distinguish the reasons for and the origins of that movement.

As an example at a different scale, consider the micro-geography of children's movement in a typical western city. The advent of mass car ownership has made a child's journey to school far more dangerous than in the past. The most likely way in which a child will die is from being hit by a car, and their likelihood of being hit by a car depends greatly on their movements (and the movements of cars). We began this section by discussing the spread of infectious diseases around the world through human migration. Micro-movements can be just as important. In Britain, childhood infections peak in the autumn, for example, after children return to school and are herded together in classrooms.

So, people change their physical location and this has an influence on the patterns of health we see, both globally and locally. Health patterns are changed because people move, and people's health is influenced by the nature of the

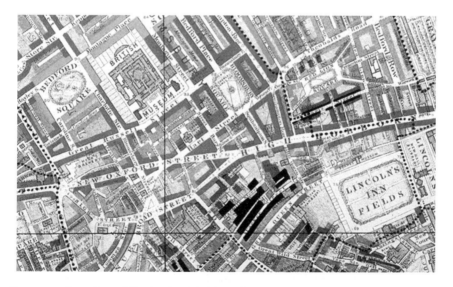

Figure 6.7 A section of Charles Booth's Map of London Poverty, 1896. The areas shaded black are the poorest areas.

moves that they make. We have analysed the results of a large cohort study – the British Household Panel Study – which suggests that much of the health divide seen in Britain today is created and maintained by a series of migrations which generally have the effect of maintaining, and sometimes increase, the health divide (for more details of this research see: Brimblecombe *et al.*, 1999 and 2000).

Socio–spatial movement

In the examples above we have attempted to separate geographical movements from social movements. This is a useful way to begin to think about the influences of movement and change on health but in reality these two aspects are rarely separate. Geographical movements are caused by, accompany and in turn cause, social change. Social change often causes, accompanies and is maintained by, geographical movements. As these changes occur in tandem they influence health and are in turn influenced by health. 'Everything' may be connected to 'everything' else, but by dissecting the various influences – even artificially presenting issues as being of places or of social groups – we can begin to see these connections. Here we show some examples of how both social and spatial movements, working together, have affected human health (see Figure 6.8).

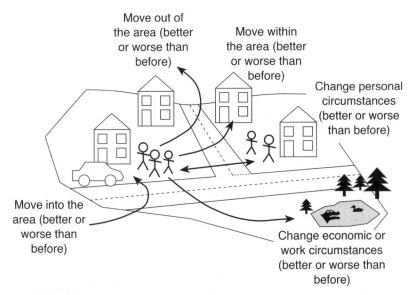

Think about how each movement could lead to better or worse health. Which of these are internal or external?

Figure 6.8 Social and spatial movements.

Class immigration

A ghetto is the product of two types of movement: immigration into a particular area and the stereotyping into a particular social group. As we have already mentioned, the original ghetto was the area of Venice where Jews were allowed to live. Both the stereotyping of people as Jewish (the creation and maintenance of a racial and religious social order) and the demarcation of the particular piece of land as a ghetto were necessary for this concentration of people to occur. Ghettos today come in many shapes and sizes but always have the feature of aligning particular social groups with particular places. Where the connection between place and identity of the resident group is weaker, the word ghetto is not used – then 'segregation' is said to have taken place.

Entire countries can have their class and geographical orders altered dramatically by large-scale immigration of particular social groups (*macro social* and *spatial* movement). Again, changes in health can be both a precursor and a consequence of such shifts. Take, for instance, the Irish Famine of the 1840s. It was the risk of poor health, the threat to life itself resulting from famine, that led so many people to leave Ireland in those years. Their emigration altered the social class system of England and the United States. In the former the Irish tended to enter near the bottom of the social hierarchy, in the latter they were more successful in entering higher up; however, in both cases they altered the system into which they arrived.

Class migration

For an example of the social and spatial interaction of movements at a more local scale think about how the gentrification of an area can result from both of these types of movements. The type of people who move into a gentrifying area tend to be richer than those who lived there before – indeed that is why it is said to be gentrifying. Moreover, they tend to move there because they are aware, perceive or anticipate that the area is gentrifying. At the same time the social status of the people who continue to live in a gentrifying community rises. The value of their homes (if they own them) increases and they become 'richer'. Other people are forced to leave the area because they can no longer afford to live there. Overall levels of health in the area are seen to improve but this improvement is a product of at least three changes: the in-migration of one group, the improved position of those who remain, and the out-migration of a poorer group who are usually also those most likely to suffer poorer health.

Take another, rather more extreme, example of the interaction of social and spatial movement. A young man is living in a rented flat in the community just described. His rent increases and at the same time he loses his job, his relationship with his partner breaks down and he begins to drink heavily. He is evicted from his flat and as he is now dependent on social security payments he cannot find another flat to rent because all the homes in the area have become too expensive for him. He finds himself spending the night with friends ('sofa surfing') but when they get fed up with him he moves to a homeless shelter, then sleeps on the streets. He then leaves the area with the hope of finding some cheap accommodation that he can afford. His social position has changed, as has his spatial location. His health, both physical and mental, is likely to have deteriorated.

The effects of health on mobility

Finally let's consider how health can affect social and spatial mobility. We begin with examples at three geographical levels:

1 *The macro scale*. We discussed in Chapter 2 how the onset of the Black Death changed entire class systems worldwide. Many would argue that AIDS is having a similar effect across much of the continent of Africa today. In the richer parts of the world improving health has altered the balance between the numbers of younger and older people – changing entire social systems. Were we to experience another influenza pandemic that killed younger people (such as that of 1918/19 which is thought to have killed as many as 20 million people) our social systems would be changed further. The growth in mental illness worldwide (or at least its recognition) will be affecting the organization of societies at the macro-level.

2 *The national scale*. The introduction of the NHS in Britain improved the health of many and to an extent narrowed gaps between social groups and places. The spread of this system of health-care management to many other countries of the world had a similar effect. If one country experiences a flood of drug imports, crime rates can quickly soar and the structure of society is changed as powers of surveillance are increased. Drugs are as much about health as about crime. Suppose that a huge anti-smoking campaign is started nationally in the country in which you live. Nicotine patches are given out freely, the price of cigarettes is doubled: what effect would this have on inequalities in health between different social classes?

3 *The individual level*. The ill effects of drink on the young man described above contributed to him becoming homeless. You may suffer from an illness while at school or university that affects your results and in turn alters your social position later in life (suffering from depression is just one very common example). Someone can be injured at work and no longer be able to earn a living. A rapid deterioration in health in your old age leads to you losing your social independence and having to move home. You are born with a disability which affects how the rest of your life pans out. We can give examples from the extreme to the trivial of how health can influence social and spatial mobility.

Although this chapter has concerned itself with the movements of people, the movements of goods, trade and services are also influential on health. Most obviously the global spread of medicine and of particular medical procedures such as immunization has a direct influence. Least obviously the global spread of profit motives and the concentration of wealth in the hands of fewer and fewer individuals has a countervailing influence. These movements of medicines and money are not independent. Some of the wealthiest people in the world enhance their wealth through their ownership of shares in pharmaceutical companies.

Finally, just as we could have gone into detail about the global spread of medicines and the concentration of profits in the last section, here we also discuss national movements of things other than people. Most clear perhaps are factors such as environmental pollution – the concentration of air pollution in particular cities or the distribution of climate and weather across a country. However, pollution is made by people – we choose how much to release and where. Similarly, the effects of climate and weather can usually be mitigated by the actions of people. People do not die particularly early of the effects of cold in Scandinavia because they build good homes and transport systems. We believe that it is the movements of people and their decisions that are most important in influencing and maintaining the geography and sociology of health.

Conclusion

Social and spatial change affects health: it affects the distribution of poor health and well-being, and people's experience of these. Moving, socially or physically, can be beneficial or detrimental to health. Which of these it turns out to be depends on the nature of the move, the individual or group who are moving, and the origin and destination.

The relationships between movement and health are complicated, but can be simplified using models and ideas to help structure the way we look at them. To simplify to a point where you can begin to understand what is going on, a particular schema or framework can be useful. As you map observations about the world onto your framework, you begin to understand more about the relationships between your observations and your ideas. Tensions between observations and frameworks are a useful means of enhancing both of them.

In this chapter we have introduced one possible framework to help us understand the different scales and types of social and spatial movement. Each researcher, writer and student should have their own schemas and frameworks within which they organize facts and stories to try to understand how the world works. There is no right and wrong way to make order out of the complexity of the world, but without making some order it is very difficult to begin to understand how it may be working. Different groups will argue passionately for different ways of viewing the world. Do not worry about that. Worry instead if they do not make their particular view explicit.

Further reading

- Willis, P. (1977) *Learning to Labour: How Working Class Kids Get Working Class Jobs.* Saxon House: Farnborough.
  This is a sociological classic that presents a detailed ethnographic study of a small group of working-class boys. Willis examines why it is that history repeats itself and children from working-class backgrounds are more than likely to end up in working-class jobs. While others see this educational and mobility 'failure' as the effect of socialization, social deprivation or unfavourable labelling by the school, Willis's work takes a different angle. He uncovers how working-class kids actually 'fail' themselves by developing cultures of resistance opposed to the school. Ask yourself whether this is plausible, and whether it is relevant today where you live.
- Berthoud, R. and Gershuny, J. (2000) *Seven Years in the Lives of British Families: Evidence on the Dynamics of Social Change from the British Household Panel Study.* The Policy Press: Bristol.
  This recent book presents empirical evidence from the British Household Panel Study which has followed the same 10,000 adults (in 5,000 households) every year between 1991 and 1997. It is about the dynamics of Britain's social and economic life – in family structures and relationships, in employment and household incomes, housing and political affiliations as well as health. Rather than looking at one point in time, this research looks at changes in people's lives, such as starting work, getting married, or falling into poverty. In some ways it is a British equivalent to an earlier US book:
- Coe, R., Duncan, G. and Hill, M. (eds) (1984) *Years of Poverty, Years of Plenty.* Institute for Social Research, University of Michigan: Ann Arbor.
- Haley, A. (1976) *Roots: The Saga of an American Family.* Dell Publishing Company: New York State.
  This book is an historical narrative of slavery in the American South. Based on research conducted over a period of years, Haley reconstructs the events that led to the enslavement of Kunte Kinte, the 'African' identified in his family lore as their founding father, and how he comes to live in America. Kinte, in his own history, becomes an allegory of the history of the millions of Africans taken forcibly to America, and of the people they became in the intervening years. The story begins in 1750 with a birth in an African village and it ends seven generations later in the United States at the funeral of a black professor.

Suggested activities

- At any one time there are at least a dozen textbooks available on the geography and sociology of health. Most have been published in the last few years although in your library you will find older books. Look at some of these 'old' and 'new' textbooks and try to determine how the authors categorized the world in order to understand it.
- Use the World Wide Web to find current major news stories that concern health in some way. Can you place these stories into the typology we have outlined above? If not, can you come up with a better way of organizing the debate in which to fit them?

180

- Consider your local area. Are there any 'ghettos'? Are there any physical barriers between areas or are the boundaries less tangible? What is the extent of movement in and out of these areas?
- Watch the films *The Full Monty* (directed by Peter Cattaneo, 20th Century Fox, 1997) and *Brassed Off* (directed by Mark Herman, Miramax, 1997). The former is the story of some down-to-earth Sheffield steelworkers who have been made redundant and who have fallen on desperate times. The latter is about how a community is affected by threatened mine closures.

References

Almond, M. (ed.) (1997) *The Times Atlas of European History*. Times Books: London.

BMJ (1999) Editor's choice. *BMJ*, 318, 10th April.

Brimblecombe, N., Dorling, D. and Shaw, M. (1999) Mortality and migration in Britain – first results from the British household panel survey. *Social Science and Medicine*, 49(7): 981–8.

Brimblecombe, N., Dorling, D. and Shaw, M. (2000) Migration and geographical inequalities in health in Britain: an exploration of the lifetime socio-economic characteristics of migrants. *Social Science and Medicine*, 50(6): 861–78.

Clarkson, T. (1817) *An essay on the slavery and commerce of the human species, particularly the African, translated from a Latin dissertation, which was honoured with the first prize in the University of Cambridge for the year 1785, with additions*. J. Phillips: London.

Davey Smith, G., Shaw, M. and Dorling, D. (1998) Shrinking areas and mortality. *The Lancet*, 352: 1139–40.

Hobsbawm, E. (1999) *Uncommon people: Resistance, Rebellion and Jazz*. The New Press: New York.

Howe, G.M. (1972) *Man, Environment and Disease in Britain: A Medical Geography of Britain Through the Ages*. David & Charles: Newton Abbot.

Thompson, E.P. (1964) *The Making of the English Working Class*. Penguin: London.

Chapter 7

Putting research into context: from cholera to good health for all

Chapter summary

In this final chapter we take an historical tour through the mapping of disease. While on one level this chapter is about how different researchers have mapped disease and mortality in different times and in different places, on another level it is about how we need to appreciate that research is conducted within different perspectives. All interpretations of the world, including this one, need to be seen as 'of their time and place'. The chapter is thus about developing thinking and being critical.

During this journey we revisit many of the topics, concepts, methods and perspectives of the preceding chapters. We reiterate the importance of an historical perspective and a sense of 'what has gone before'. We see again elements of the social and spatial patterning of health and illness. We think once more about how diseases can be measured and mapped and about the patterns of health inequalities that we see as a consequence. Issues of composition and context, migration and mobility are never far from the frame.

Through this we hope to convince you that 'the answer' is not always out there. It is constantly being created and recreated by people from all walks of life, expressed in all kinds of ways, at different times and in different places – we aim to put research into context.

We finish by outlining the key messages that we hope this book has conveyed.

Introduction

Before we begin to consider some specific historical examples of the mapping of disease we shall briefly sketch what we are aiming to achieve in this concluding chapter. We hope to illustrate, by exploring a themed collection of examples, the following: what changes in research and what stays the same, how views of disease are altered and how researchers come to use particular techniques to study particular problems, and how all of this work is affected by the social, spatial and temporal context of the topic and of the studies themselves. As we journey through a century and a half of the mapping of disease we want you to think about influences on the work of the researchers we feature, including when and where they were working. How might they have conducted their work differently had they been able to access all of the ideas we have presented in this book? Taking this a step further, to what extent are the ideas presented in this book contingent on the time and place in which *we* are writing? To what extent are we as authors dominated by the country we come from (Britain) and by the research that has dominated the time we have worked in (the 1990s)? How much can we learn from the past to help us understand our limitations and to see how limited our work may appear in a few decades' time? It is these critical thoughts that we would like you to carry with you as we take you through a version (*our* version) of the history of disease mapping.

The origins of modern disease mapping

Let's start with the advent of disease mapping. More than any other disease in the eighteenth century it was cholera that provoked the demand for an understanding of how people's location and their health are related. Death from cholera infection is a particularly painful process, as the film recommended in Chapter 2, *The Horseman on the Roof,* depicts. Outbreaks of cholera occurred at the same time as the nineteenth-century revolution in thinking about the nature of society, which makes cholera an ideal case study for understanding how people began to link the geography of a disease to the workings of a society, in a coherent fashion.

Figure 7.1 shows one of the earliest chloropleth maps of disease ever drawn. It was drawn by Rothenburg and it depicts the 1832 epidemic of cholera in Hamburg. Cartographic historian Arthur Robinson has speculated that this map inspired the creation of many others. In particular, he says that

Looking back in time can help
us see better in the present

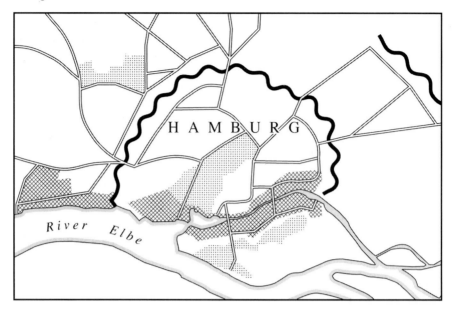

Figure 7.1 Rothenburg's 1836 map of cholera in Hamburg in 1832. (Hatched areas mark cholera outbreaks. Darker areas show where the epidemic was most intense.)
Source: Robinson (1982).

'Rothenburg's map was redrawn and included in the report of the British General Board of Health on the epidemic of cholera which for the second time visited Britain in 1848–49' (Robinson, 1982: 171). It is interesting to note that the map, which showed the prevalence of disease and was apparently influential in cartographic circles, was said to have been largely ignored by that Health Board.

A second major disease, which grew further in importance after the eighteenth century, was influenza. In the same year that cholera was being mapped in Hamburg (Germany), an influenza epidemic was occurring in Glasgow (Scotland). A map of the geography of that 1832 influenza epidemic was produced by the inmates of a 'lunatic' asylum, a task given to them by a doctor, mainly as a means to occupy their time (Cliff and Haggett, 1988). This was one of the earliest examples of disease mapping in Britain and the fact that this was a task allotted to 'lunatics' shows how little value was placed on this technique at that time. Our trip through history thus starts at a time when the mapping of disease was on the verge of being taken seriously. It is worth asking yourself why – from such humble beginnings and in a matter of a few years – did this technique became a mainstream method for understanding of illness?

Later in the nineteenth century the value of mapping disease patterns was more widely recognized as specific epidemiological breakthroughs were attributed to the insight gained from plotting the spatial patterns of disease. Most often cited is a map of the distribution of deaths from the 1848 cholera epidemic in London (England) which, so the tale goes, inspired the removal of the handle of the water pump at the centre of a cluster of dots on the map, resulting in the curtailing of the epidemic (Snow, 1854). The map, shown in Figure 7.2, came to be seen as having a definitive influence on the Board of Health that met to address the epidemic. However, just how important was the map to the halting of the epidemic, compared with the way that the role of the map is often presented? This story unravels in the following sections.

Maps can be wonderful things but they can also be problematic. People have an amazing ability to discern patterns in maps – even when there is really none to be seen. Of course, the converse of this 'problem' is that the human eye is an excellent tool for identifying weak patterning when it does exist. Often 'clusters' seen on maps are artefacts of the way the maps have been drawn, how much physical space is represented, what features the maps include.

Before reading further, look at Snow's map and ask yourself what is really being shown here? If you were presented with a map such as this showing a modern illness what questions would you ask? Maps of epidemic diseases can be viewed like news pictures of a dramatic event. The maps, after all, are telling dramatic stories. You should always ask yourself what is *not* being shown in a map while looking at what *is* there – just as you should do with a television news report. In particular, look around the edge of the map. Ask why it ends where

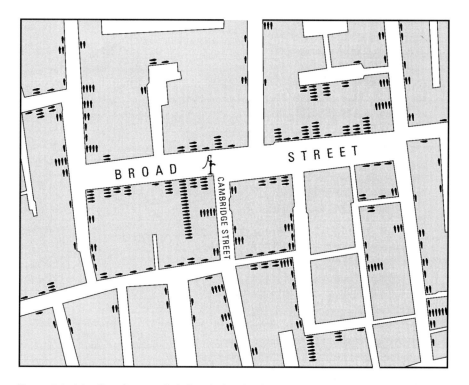

Figure 7.2 John Snow's map of cholera in London in 1854.

Source: Cliff and Haggett (1988).

it does. For instance, maps of diseases are often centred on the point the author thinks is of most importance. Figure 7.2 shows the central section of John Snow's map of deaths from cholera in Soho. Your eye is automatically drawn to the pump in the centre of the map, particularly by the very high number of deaths at the intersection of Cambridge and Broad Streets. Had John Snow shown all of London in his map he would have discovered an even greater concentration of deaths just south of the river Thames, as shown in Figure 7.3. This concentration would have moved location again had Snow used an isodemographic base map (one in which the space on the page is proportional to the size of the population), as shown in Figure 7.4. But such maps had not been invented by then. As you draw the map in different ways, the pattern that your map shows can change too. In its infancy, in nineteenth-century London, medical map-making was blind to these distortions.

The fact that John Snow's map is not a particularly good example of medical mapping would not be worthy of so much discussion here were it not for the fact that it has continuously been presented as a prime exemplar (recently, for example, by a famous author on mapping and visualization – Edward Tufte,

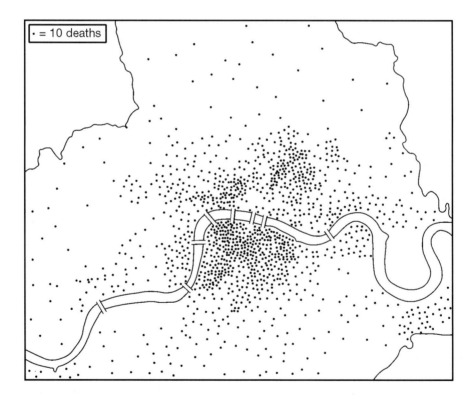

Figure 7.3 Cholera deaths in London in 1849. All human disease mapping of this kind is extremely misleading.

Source: redrawn from Cliff and Haggett (1988), Figure 1.3B.

186

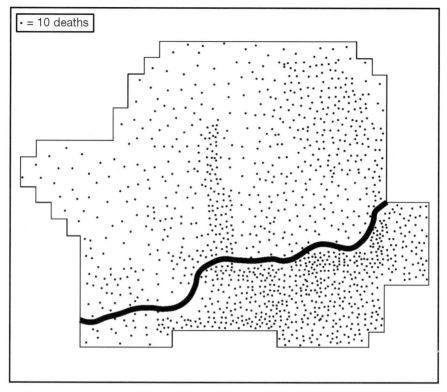

Figure 7.4 Cholera deaths in London in 1849 drawn on an equal population cartogram, showing the true density of cases.

Source: redrawn from Cliff and Haggett (1988) Figure 1.18D, with river added.

1997). The story goes that by mapping the disease, noticing a cluster centred around the Broad Street water pump and then removing the pump handle, Snow defeated the cholera epidemic in that area. Many people have subsequently declared that Snow led the way in medical map-making. The next section explains how this famous map was not the means by which the source of cholera could have been discovered and, more importantly, how the construction of the map ignored the social events of its times. We continue to focus on this example because it teaches us valuable lessons about how to view, evaluate and judge social research.

Putting the Broad Street pump into context

Following the cholera epidemic in South London in 1848, Dr John Snow published *On the Mode of Communication of Cholera* in 1849. Snow's work provided the data that led to the conclusion that cholera was carried through polluted drinking water. However, the first edition of Snow's book did *not* include any maps (Rip *et al.*, 1998). It was not 'the map' which convinced the authorities of the time that cholera cases were clustered. In the second edition of Snow's book the now famous map of the 1854 outbreak in Soho *was* included (see Figure 7.2) showing the apparent clustering of cholera deaths around the Broad Street pump, but it was not (as so often claimed) the drawing of that map which led to the identification of the cluster. That Snow did not use his map to identify the Broad Street pump as the conduit for the Soho cholera outbreak is obvious from the map itself, and from a reading of Snow's work. The map is *centred* on the pump. The pump was seen as the cause before the map was even drawn. The pump was not identified from the map, the map was drawn as evidence to corroborate a theory. In addition, it is well known (and even one of the enthusiastic accounts of the role of the map reports) that the number of deaths from cholera was falling a week *before* the pump handle was removed. Perpetuation of the myth that Snow's map solved the cholera mystery reinforces the idea that dot density mapping is 'the' way to find clusters of disease. In reality the map was not used to identify the clustering or cause of cholera in 1854 and if you were trying to identify such a cause or cluster today, this is not the kind of map you should draw.

A century and a half later Snow's work still raises interesting questions. Was it specifically and only the water in the Broad Street pump that was contaminated? Why were the *environmental* causes of disease of such interest to Snow, given the huge range of *social* inequalities that were being identified at that time (Chadwick, 1842; Engels, 1844)? We should also think about the social and historical context of the time. We could argue that it was the 1848 worldwide cholera epidemic and the uprisings of that year in Berlin, Paris, Vienna, Sicily, Milan, Naples, Parma, Rome, Warsaw, Prague and Budapest that were the historical companions of the first Public Health Act in Britain. The act created the General Board of Health that year, empowered to establish local boards of health to manage water supply and sewerage (Krieger *et al.*, 1997). These events, along with many other factors, led to improved living conditions in Britain. It can be argued that changes such as this were the true precursors to the removal of the pump handle in Soho five years later, rather than the mapping of cholera. We often like to think that science leads the way, but often it is *social* changes that are predominant. In this case, science *confirmed* the idea that diseases could be spread through dirty water – only after social changes to improve the general living conditions of the working population were well under way.

This debate has resonance today, when a report of a cluster of half a dozen deaths in a dozen years around a power station will result in far more public interest, research funding and publications than does the knowledge that tens of thousands of people die prematurely every year in Britain due to relative poverty. The deaths of people in an earthquake will often make headlines, but the many thousands of deaths that occur in the same area over a sustained period of time – but due to poverty and poor sanitary conditions – will receive very little mention. We can understand earthquakes, we can blame them on an 'act of god' or the movement of tectonic plates according to our view of the world. Pollution from a power station we can visualize, even if we cannot actually see it. We can imagine how living with pollution might harm us. The workings of societies that promote the interests of a few over those of the majority are harder to see on a day-to-day basis. It sounds like a cliché, but society really does kill many more people in an 'everyday' way than disasters or point sources of pollution – it's just not newsworthy.

From a different sociological and geographical perspective the story of the Broad Street pump can be read another way. It was poverty, and the commensurate overcrowding, exhaustion and infirmity that it caused, which led to the concentration of susceptible people in this part of Soho (Dorling, 1998). It also led to them remaining there after the most affluent had fled. This is *not* the story presented in popular retellings of John Snow's tale. In Edward Tufte's book on 'visual explanations' (1997) Tufte reports (but did not remark upon) Snow's comment that '[P]ersons in furnished lodgings left first, then other lodgers went away, leaving their furniture to be sent for' (Snow, 1855, in Tufte, 1997: 27). Those in furnished lodgings left first because they had the resources to do so, not because they were not worried about their furniture. Think back to Chapter 6 where we discussed the importance of mobility in determining patterns of disease. Here we have an example of very short-term geographical mobility affecting which social groups were most vulnerable to disease. Next think back to Chapter 5 and the importance of context. In this case, in what circumstances were these people living? How were these people represented by Snow's map? Tufte admits that 'the big problem is that dot maps fail to take into account the number of people living in an area' (1997: 35). Cliff and Haggett (1988) have subsequently shown how Snow's data could be re-mapped on an isodemographic map base (see Figures 7.3 and 7.4). Their maps show a very different picture.

An interesting addendum to this story is that Tufte himself used the first edition of John Snow's work, which does not actually contain Snow's maps, only his text. Tufte thus re-drew Snow's map from a later version of his text, and it is this version that has been widely reproduced, not Snow's original map. Many redrawn versions of the map in numerous textbooks fail to reproduce important elements of the original. This might partly explain some misinterpretation of the story and it is a good warning to the reader to try to return to original work wherever possible.

The persistent relationship between health and place

As we learn about the interplay of social inequalities and disease perhaps we should compare the maps of disease distribution to maps of social conditions. An interesting alternative to Snow's map is one published exactly one hundred years later, plotting the distribution of poliomyelitis on a cartogram of London (Taylor, 1955; see Figure 7.5). This map was far cruder than Snow's and did not have the same impact on health as that with which Snow is credited. It is, however, an example of a working General Practitioner mapping in novel ways and attempting to understand the geography, causes and consequences of the diseases of their day. Taylor was studying the distribution of polio in 1947 and his map identified the highest rates to be in Shoreditch (a poor area) and the lowest rates in Islington and areas around Hampstead (richer areas). Rates are lowest where the heights of the bars within the borough rectangles are lowest, irrespective of width. Most of today's epidemics are similarly geographically patterned from poor to rich areas although infectious and viral diseases that spread through sewage are no longer epidemic in the West (as we noted in Chapter 4). In 1991, Shoreditch was home to the highest proportion of people in low-paid work in Britain: 39 per cent of its economically active residents were in unskilled or semi-skilled manual labour (compared with just 11 per cent in Hampstead, one of the lowest rates in the country). Shoreditch also has the highest premature mortality rate among adults in Britain (Dorling, 1997: 48).

Snow's story of the widow living in Hampstead who died because she had water delivered from the Broad Street pump tells us as much about the social geography of London in the past as it does about cholera: 'A niece, who was on a visit to this lady, also drank of the water; she returned to her residence, in a high and healthy part of Islington, was attacked with cholera, and died also. There was no cholera at this time, either at West End [Hampstead] or in the neighbourhood where the niece died' (Snow on Fraser's report in Tufte, 1997: 32). The geographical contours of inequalities in health in London have changed little over time.

Exactly a century and a half after the cholera epidemic that began this story, homeless people found on the streets of London are dying (albeit in much lower numbers) in much the same geographical distribution as those who died from cholera in Snow's time. In fact, among London's homeless population, the average age of death is 42, very close to the average age of death for the whole population of England and Wales a century and a half ago (Shaw and Dorling, 1998). Comparing maps of cholera deaths in 1848 with deaths from homelessness in 1998 shows how mapping can help understand how slowly the processes that drive human geographies of ill health actually change. Cholera killed people most in Oxford, for instance, in very similar places to where the homeless hostels are now situated in that city (see Chapter 4, example 3, p. 121).

What should we learn from this tale? The belief that 'taking a handle off a pump' can solve society's ills continues today. We can see now that this area of London has continued to be a focus for disease and premature mortality. Early epidemiology and public health measures managed to control the infectious diseases that were concentrated there, but in time these were replaced by other causes of death and no doubt they will continue to be so. Today, homelessness focuses illness and death in and around the same streets. We continue to make great strides in tackling individual diseases through medicine, but medical understanding has not helped to change the socio-spatial patterns of good and poor health over the last 150 years very much at all. Would John Snow be shocked to hear that people still die of poverty on the streets of Soho,

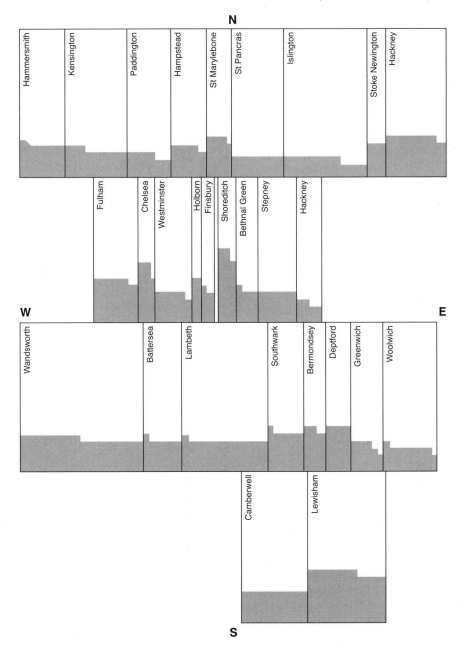

Figure 7.5 Taylor's map of polio in London in 1955.

Source: Taylor (1955). Note: Taylor used square paper to draw this diagram by hand – hence the 'steps' in some of the bar charts.

even though we now employ techniques in medicine that he could never have dreamt of?

Old and new ways of mapping disease _____

Disease mapping has been strongly influenced, not surprisingly, by the history of diseases themselves – as the phenomena we study change, so do our methods for studying them. Figure 7.6 shows the prevalence of six major causes of death in England and Wales since the publication of Snow's map of cholera. Infectious diseases now account for a tiny fraction of deaths in rich countries. Other causes of death (such as suicide) are declining for some age–sex groups but not for others. When some causes of death decline in relative importance some necessarily have to rise. Cancers, for instance, account for an increasing proportion of deaths. As diseases rise in the proportion of total mortality that they account for, they become more interesting to researchers. In terms of mapping these contemporary diseases the analysis of point patterns in relation to particular locations is still a major issue. However, with chronic diseases such as cancer the patterns that are obtained are usually less clear than those seen in outbreaks of infectious disease. More importantly, it is increasingly accepted that more abstract factors, like 'social inequality', can themselves lie behind particular patterns of disease (as we saw in Chapter 5). In turn, these require more 'abstract' mappings for proper study.

One of the traditional mapping techniques is *chloropleth* mapping, in which areas on a map are shaded according to statistics about the population of each area (see Figure 7.1 and Chapter 3). Mapping areas and shading them according to their standardized mortality ratios is one common form of chloropleth mapping in medical geography or sociology. Another traditional technique is to map points, each of which marks the incidences of disease. Colour can be used with both these techniques, of course. In addition, a variety of symbols can be

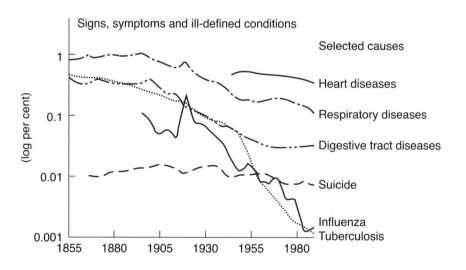

Figure 7.6 Change in causes of death in England and Wales, 1855–1990.

Source: Dorling (1995, Fig. 5.21).

used in point mapping, rather than just simple points. For instance, circles can be coloured or segmented to highlight different features of a disease and they can be sized in proportion to incidence or population. When these proportional symbols are used this technique begins to merge with *isodemographic mapping*.

We have already mentioned isodemographic mapping here (Figure 7.4) and in Chapter 3. We shall now take a closer look at its evolution. This type of mapping indicates a different way of thinking about the distribution of disease; in a way it marks a coming together of the notion of place *and* (groups of) people. Chloropleth and point maps portray how diseases vary across *land*, but diseases also vary across populations. Quite simply, where there are more people there is more possibility for the incidence of disease. We should thus take account of the distribution of the population at risk of a particular disease (the number of people 'available' to be ill or to die) before mapping its distribution. One way in which this can be done is to use a map projection which draws every area *in proportion to the number of people* living in that area, hence the term isodemographic, which literally means 'equal people'. Isodemographic maps are also called *cartograms* and are used for many purposes, though disease mapping is perhaps one of their more established uses (political mapping is *the* most established use).

Figure 7.7 shows one of the earliest examples of a cartogram designed 'for epidemiological purposes' (Wallace, 1926: 1023). Figure 7.7(a) is a conventional map of the counties in Iowa State and (b) is an equal population cartogram upon which coloured pins were placed to show the locations of 'notifiable diseases' (which we discussed in Chapter 3). The square in the middle of the cartogram is the populous Des Moines city in Polk County. The map was used to study the introduction of a vaccine which was supposed to prevent colds.

The designer of the Iowa cartogram was a doctor working in the state department of health. Many researchers have been struck by the idea that they could learn more about disease through mapping it in non-traditional ways. As stated above, the first cartogram of London was an 'epidemiological map' produced by a doctor working for the then London County Council Department of Public Health (Taylor, 1955). That early cartogram (Figure 7.5) contained crosses drawn in the borough rectangles to show the incidence of polio during the 1947 epidemic. Here we have replaced the crosses by bars in redrawing the figure. Since the rectangles were each drawn with the same height, their widths are proportional to population as well as their areas. As we have already noted, the borough with the highest rate of polio (and hence the tallest column of crosses in the figure) was Shoreditch.

Why should a doctor working in Iowa in 1926, and one studying completely independently in London in 1955, come up with the same technique? Before these dates only a handful of cartograms had been produced and none of these concerned patterns of health. It is also very unlikely that these doctors had seen each other's maps or any earlier examples. The answer perhaps lies in the *timing* of these maps. By the start of the twentieth century people were beginning to

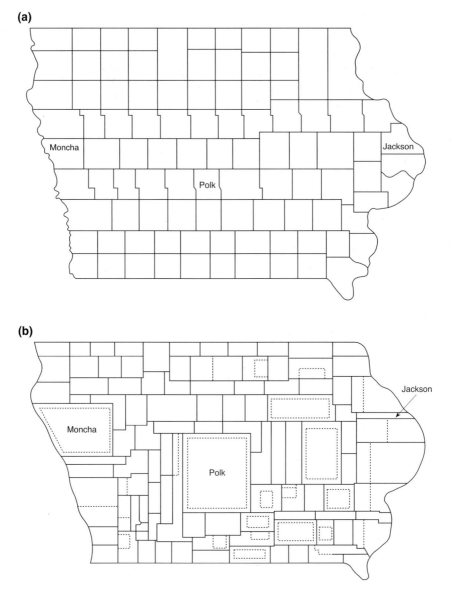

Figure 7.7 The use of a 'cold vaccine' in Iowa counties.
Source: Wallace (1926).

think of disease in terms of the populations it affected – rather than concentrating on the disease itself. The two maps are interesting not only because of the particular local patterns of disease that they mapped but also, perhaps more so, because they mark a shift in perspective – a different way of seeing the world.

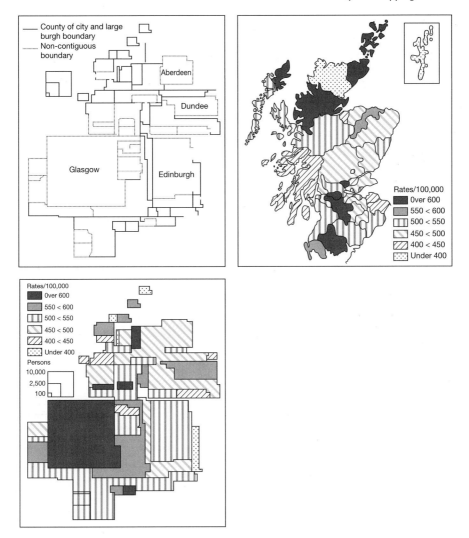

Figure 7.8 Forster's mapping of mortality rates in Scotland.

Source: Forster (1966). © BMJ Publishing Group

A decade after Taylor's cartograms of polio in London the first cartograms showing national disease distributions were produced (Forster, 1966). Forster produced maps of mortality for Scotland and constructed (by hand) a cartogram for each of eight age–sex groups. Figure 7.8 shows the cartogram which depicted the mortality of women in Scotland aged 45 to 54 for 1959–63. Forster concluded that a national series of cartograms should be produced for all age–sex groups for use in epidemiological studies. This work was never done, and it is debatable whether such an exact mapping base is needed in most studies. A single, well-constructed, cartogram of the whole population will usually suffice to uncover all but the most subtle of patterns in general mortality or morbidity. A single cartogram was used later by Howe as we discuss below, but first what did Forster's new maps show?

Interest in all-cause mortality (rather than from specific diseases) increased greatly from the 1960s onwards. These maps, showing the distribution of all-cause mortality in Scotland, uncovered a pattern whereby illness was shown to be concentrated in the poorer cities, and most obviously Glasgow. By drawing the maps in proportion to the population, Forster highlighted just how important Glasgow was to this pattern, because Glasgow is the major centre of population in Scotland. On the conventional map of Scotland shown in Figure 7.8 a relatively sparsely populated area of the Scottish Borders dominates the map as having the highest rate and largest expanse of space on the paper.

It is important to realize that these first national cartograms of disease were drawn only 30–40 years ago. Before then no one had 'seen' the clear picture of mortality in Scotland that they presented. Although tables of figures had been produced and the highest and lowest mortality areas listed for more than a century, there is something qualitatively different between reading a table of figures and seeing a pattern in front of your eyes. The juxtaposition of poor areas and rich areas, the repetition of patterns across a map, similarities with other well-known distributions – seeing these things on a page (or screen) steers your thoughts towards the underlying issues in a way that looking at a list of numbers simply cannot. The cartograms also force the reader to concentrate on what affects the greatest numbers of people.

To continue our historical tour of the mapping of disease *A National Atlas of Disease Mortality in the United Kingdom* was published in 1963 under the auspices of the Royal Geographical Society, although the atlas did not contain any cartograms. However, a revised edition was published a few years later which made copious use of a 'demographic base map' (Howe, 1970: 95). It is interesting to note that when the revised edition was being prepared, the president of the Society was Dudley Stamp. Stamp believed that 'the fundamental tool for geographical analysis is undoubtedly the map or, perhaps more correctly, the cartogram' (Stamp, 1962: 135). In the cartogram which was used in the revised national atlas (Figure 7.9), squares represented urban areas while diamonds were used to show statistics for rural districts. A stylized coastline was placed around the symbols, which were all drawn with their areas in proportion to the populations at risk from the particular disease being shown.

Howe's national cartogram was used to display the distribution of standardized mortality ratios (explained in Chapter 3) between 1959 and 1963 from specific causes of death, as well as all causes of death, for both men and women. High rates were seen in northern districts and some Inner London boroughs (including Shoreditch, which was highlighted *again*). Extremely high rates in central Scotland were particularly noticeable as were the low rates in the districts surrounding London. At the extremes, these maps showed that an average man living in Salford was 50 per cent more likely to die in a typical year than his

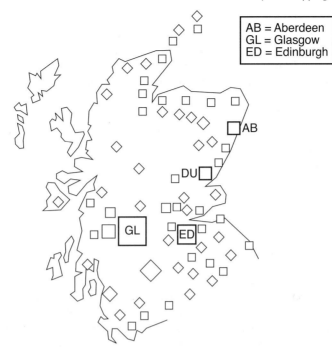

Figure 7.9 Howe's cartogram for mapping disease in the UK (only Scotland shown).
Source: Howe (1970).

counterpart in Bournemouth (Howe, 1970: 98). Both these areas appear quite small on a 'normal' map, and thus fail to get the attention they deserve. The pattern for women was very similar to that for men.

Looking at Howe's maps and comparing them with those produced by Forster a decade earlier (see Figure 7.8) generates many interesting and important questions about what drives geographical and social health inequalities. What Howe achieved was to produce a series of images of the spatial distribution of disease; these were subsequently seen by many students (including the authors of this book) and the rapidly expanding cohort of researchers coming into the field. He presented the patterns that led others to ask the questions of how these patterns were created and maintained.

Why was it that these types of image should have emerged in the 1960s? Research is always embedded in its particular time and place. The social changes in the 1960s marked a change in the way that people approached many aspects of life, including research – thinking became more critical and imaginative. In sociology this meant a turn towards qualitative research, whereas in geography there were new developments in the application of quantitative techniques. Developments in computing meant that they could be used to draw simple maps. More generally, and more importantly, this was a time when researchers not only turned to new techniques but they began to question the nature of the societies they were living in with greater intensity.

Point mapping a century on: a return to clusters

Let us turn now to some of the technological developments that were creeping into medical geography as quantitative techniques became more accepted. Isodemographic mapping is now used to study the prevalence and distribution of individual cases of a disease. In this sense we have come full circle from Snow's day. Figure 7.10 shows an example of when this mapping began, again in the 1960s. Figure 7.10(a) shows the distribution of cases of Wilm's tumour, a childhood cancer, identified in New York State between 1958 and 1962, drawn upon an equal land area map. Apparent clusters of cases have been marked on the map (Levison and Haddon, 1965: 56). In Figure 7.10(b) the same cases are drawn upon an equal population cartogram and the apparent clusters can be seen to have been quite evenly dispersed across the population. The same process has been used in Figure 7.11 to illustrate how cases of *Salmonella* food poisoning occurring in Arkansas in 1974 were not unduly clustered in Pulaski county (Dean, 1976).

After the 1970s researchers turned their attention to developing cartograms automatically for identifying clusters of disease and we give examples of this below. A major problem with using population cartograms to map and identify clusters of disease is that the choice of which areas are physically closest each other – on the page, or screen, of the cartogram – can be quite arbitrary. How you choose to draw the map can affect the results of your research. When we draw a cartogram that represents something such as population size, the physical shape and location of places on the map become distorted. This means that it is perfectly possible to plot incidences of one particular disease on three different types of (equally 'correct') population cartogram and see three different parts of the country with an apparently dense cluster of cases. This would be true regardless of whether the clusters were to be identified by eye or by statistical procedures; the different base maps would result in different results emerging. Using a computer algorithm to create the 'best' base map automatically removes some of this bias, but does not eliminate it – for instance, you still have the choice of deciding which algorithm is 'best'.

Science, 'truth' and maps

That there are choices to be made over designing base maps is a fine example of how (all) science which claims to be telling a 'true' story, or providing 'an answer' to a question, is often only presenting one 'version' of the truth. A scientific procedure or test tells us only what it was designed to see, not what *can be seen*. This idea, that there is no single 'true answer' as to whether a disease is

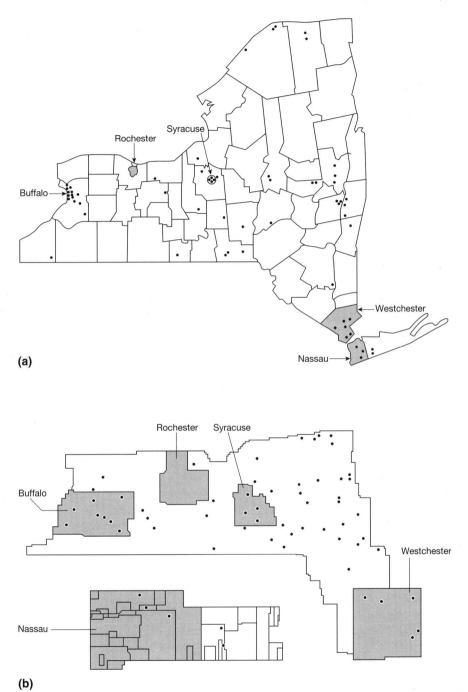

Figure 7.10 Levison and Haddon's mapping of Wilm's tumour.

Source: Levison and Haddon (1965).

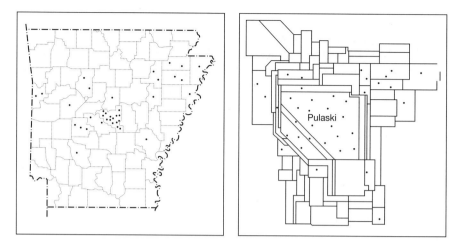

Figure 7.11 Dean's map and cartogram of Salmonella.

Source: Dean (1976).

clustered is challenging for those who would like hard and fast answers and believe that 'the truth is out there'. How clustered does a disease have to be for it to qualify as a true 'cluster'? One way to address this problem is to approach your research question with a variety of tools or tests. A group of researchers at the University of California, Berkeley, for example, developed a computer program for identifying incidences of disease (Selvin *et al.*, 1984). The algorithm was used to produce the cartogram of San Francisco county in Figure 7.12 where apparent clusters of disease were shown to be illusory (Selvin *et al.*, 1988: 217). Application of the method to another California county did provide evi-

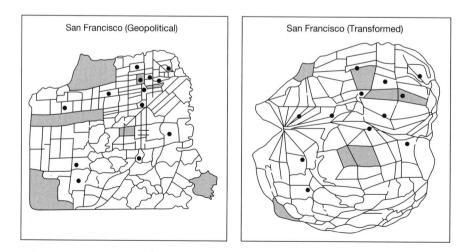

Figure 7.12 Cartograms of San Francisco: cancers and leukaemia.

Source: Selvin *et al.* (1988).

dence of some clustering of high cancer rates near oil refineries (Selvin *et al.*, 1987). But each of these pictures is a different version of the truth. The fact that they have been created by computer algorithm rather than drawn by hand does not necessarily make them more valid. The 'truth' can still easily be contested by other researchers using other techniques.

Today, mapping of disease patterns is becoming increasingly common owing to the proliferation of computers and mapping software. However, much of this software was designed to produce general maps of any subject and is often more appropriate for the mapping of land use or the distribution of points in physical space than it is for mapping health. Over most of the course of the last century, doctors, public health officials and researchers discovered and rediscovered that traditional maps often do not provide the best means of looking for patterns of disease. Our journey ends with an example of our own work, which puts much of what we have discussed above into practice.

Mapping the social aspects of health

In Chapter 3 (Research Example 1, page 78) we described a piece of research that tried to account for the changing geography of mortality in Britain during the 1980s and 1990s. For that work population cartograms of Britain were produced. Figure 3.9 showed the amount of change in premature mortality that needed to be explained between the two decades. In Chapter 3 we were mainly interested in how the statistics were calculated. Here we want you to think about how choosing this type of map to depict those statistics was a conscious decision that reflected the researchers' view of the world and that portrayed the data in a way that would have been very different had a conventional map be drawn. We know it was a very deliberate and conscious choice because we were the researchers who made the choice. That choice was made possible only because of the work which had gone on before in progressing mapping methods in medical geography. Figure 3.10 showed where the changes in mortality could not be accounted for by changes in compositional factors (age, sex, social class and employment status). Had a traditional map been used then the large swathe of unexplained high mortality in central Glasgow would be hardly visible.

The importance of cartogram mapping was further discussed in Chapter 3 (Figures 3.9 and 3.10) where we referred to it in order to open up the context/composition debate. However, the research that produced these maps took the process a step further – rather than just mapping the patterns of the recent past, it looked forward to a possible future, asking what might happen if certain policy goals were achieved. These policy goals were: if full employment were reached, if child poverty were eliminated and if there was a mild redistribution of wealth in Britain. The cartogram in Figure 7.13 shows where we think most lives would be saved if these policy aims were accomplished. On a conventional map of Britain the effect would be far less dramatic – as most lives would be saved in the places that take up least of the paper (where population density is

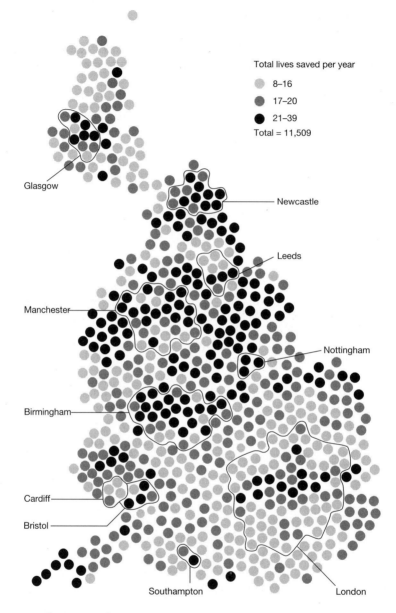

Figure 7.13 Cartogram of preventable death in Britain.
Source: Mitchell *et al.* (2000).

highest). How researchers choose to map their results is thus as important as deciding what research questions to ask and how to go about collecting and analysing data. How you approach these different elements of the research process reflects how you see the world and what you have learnt about it from work which has gone before yours.

Figure 7.13 shows where improvements in health could be achieved in one country if governments really begin to move towards their oft-stated aim of ensuring good health for all. We believe that to achieve this they need to address many other problems in society that are tangential to health and that are still not fully realized to be 'health problems'. Childhood poverty, mass unemployment and the unequal distribution of wealth are just three of these. The map shows what effect we believe addressing these problems could have on the distribution of poor health in the future. We have come a long way from mapping the repercussions of cholera, to mapping the repercussions of the way in which we organize our lives – society. However, in much of the world cholera still kills very many people early in their lives. It is a constant concern after natural disasters and in refugee camps created by wars and other human-made disasters. In some ways we have not come very far at all.

Concluding thoughts

In this final chapter we have taken a brief historical tour through the mapping of disease, focusing not only on the various methods employed, but on how different researchers have approached this issue differently – they have thought about things in different ways. We have emphasized how it is important to put research into context – in terms of time and place. We have deliberately tried not to present the most recent advances in research as the best; instead we have picked examples of innovative research from the last century and a half and tried to place this work within the context of the changing times and thinking of the place in which it was done. We have chosen this approach in order to make several points:

- Not all the 'best' research is new research.
- What is 'best' is a matter of opinion.

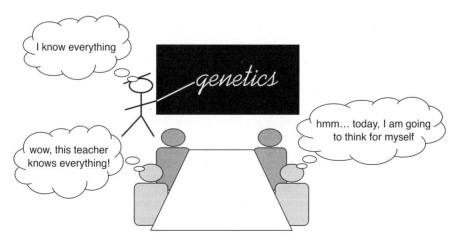

Question what you are taught, read what you can, seek a variety of opinions

- Not all techniques which purport to be 'new' are actually that 'new'.
- At different times researchers prioritize different research questions; the *subject* of research (such as the type of disease deemed important to study) changes through time.
- The *methods* of enquiry also change and develop over time.
- Sometimes two areas of study develop separately, when they are actually in effect looking at the same thing. Researchers have often found spatial patterns that are social but have not realized that, and vice versa. This is why communication between different fields of research is so important.

The story told in this chapter is, on the surface, a story of data visualization – how people first tried to draw maps of the diseases that were of most importance to their time and place, what influenced those maps and how the mapping itself changed. However, underlying this simple story of mapping is the story of rapidly changing societies – both in the wider world and within the research community.

In the nineteenth century research was very much a lone activity. Almost always it was wealthy men, working largely alone, who produced scholarly works on particular events. Throughout the twentieth century, research moved into universities and other institutions and came to be produced and published in particular ways. At the same time there was growing realization that the causes underlying patterns of disease were wider and more complex than a single 'medical' or 'social' model.

However, we would argue that by the end of the twentieth century a great deal of research has *not* learnt the lessons of the last one hundred and fifty years – that the organization of society and the distribution of health are intrinsically connected. We suspect that the failure to make proper connections between society and health are partly a result of how 'health' is taught to people whose job it is to cure illness and deal with its consequences. By concentrating on 'coping with' and 'curing' illness rather than 'understanding and altering society', medicine and society continue to remain too far apart. A large part of this misunderstanding comes from how 'health' is currently taught – as 'medicine'. As researchers we are almost all guilty of not looking enough at what creates and maintains good health – partly because there is little precedent for this, partly because it would be difficult to get funding to do such work.

In this book we have tried to introduce the reader to the breadth and depth of issues, findings and techniques which constitute a quantitative approach to studying health in society and space. In Chapter 2 we took an historical perspective on social and spatial aspects of health. In Chapter 3 the basic concepts of modern health and disease mapping and measurement were introduced. In Chapter 4 we looked at social and spatial patterns in health, from the global to the local level. In Chapter 5 we looked more closely at discussion of the effects of contextual and compositional factors. In Chapter 6 we added the concepts of migration and mobility to the discussion of how patterns of good and poor health are created and maintained. In this chapter we have returned to an historical theme and traced the development of health mapping in order to show

how science itself takes place in the context of time and place – as does the 'science' which tries to understand it.

Our account of the history of mapping is obviously, like all the chapters in the book, a selective one. We have presented you with one view – *our* view – of the crossroads of medical geography and sociology and have combined them in ways that we think make sense – but you may not. No one can understand everything – no one can grasp the history of all the places listed in Box 7.1, nor the nature of each disease mentioned, nor all the different ways in which each could have been studied, let alone the full context in which all this work occurred. What you can do, however, is gain an overview of such work, look outside your particular area of study, have an eye for what else was taking place at the same time and what else is being done now. Think and work critically.

What we would like you to take away from having read this book is first and foremost the idea that in health research, nothing is certain, much is still poorly understood and very few issues are actually 'new' or exclusively about *either* health *or* society/space. We would like you to understand our argument that the medical model for the understanding of health is grossly inadequate when used alone, but that the study of health in the social sciences needs to avoid narrow geographical, historical or sociological accounts. Instead we need to look across disciplines. You will find as you read more that many books and papers try to steer their readers towards particular established accounts of the world, towards a view that is dominant in one academic discipline or another and subsequently towards either reading the medical *or* sociological *or* geographical literature. Academia tends to shy away from novels, newspaper and films and encourages more formal study via the belief that there is an answer 'out there' if only you read and understand enough.

'The answer' is not always 'out there'. It is constantly being created and recreated by people from all walks of life, expressed in all kinds of ways, at different times and in different places. Everyone who has something to say about health has been influenced by the (relatively short) time they have had to learn, by their

---

Box 7.1 Our examples of the mapping of disease, 1832–2000

Hamburg	Cholera	1832
Glasgow	Influenza	1832
London	Cholera	1848
Iowa	Cold	1926
London	Polio	1955
New York	Wilm's tumour	1965
Scotland	All-cause mortality	1966
UK	Many-cause mortality	1970
Arkansas	*Salmonella*	1976
San Francisco	Cancers	1984
Britain	Preventable death	2000

social ties and the places they grew up in and by the particular ways in which they were taught to think. We have presented you with our thoughts and ideas and some possible ways for you to take your own ideas forward. Whether or not you like our ideas, we encourage you to search out others. After you have done that, why not try to develop your own, new and hopefully more complete understanding of health, place and society?

Further reading

We encourage you to read original historical sources. The following reader presents extracts from a range of thinkers, including: Thomas Malthus, William Farr, Edwin Chadwick, Karl Marx, Richard Titmuss and Aneurin Bevan. (Read the books written or edited by us only if you want to know how our thinking has developed!)

- Davey Smith, G., Dorling, D. and Shaw, M. (2001) *Poverty, Inequality and Health in Britain – 1800–2000: A Reader*. The Policy Press: Bristol.

If you interested in how the future might be read:

- Wagar, W. (1999) (3rd edn) *A Short History of the Future*. University of Chicago Press: Chicago.
- WHO (1998) *The World Health Report 1998: Life in the Twenty-first Century: A Vision for All*. WHO: Geneva.
  This report considers what will life be like in the twenty-first century. Will the world continue to grow healthier, with ever more diseases conquered by scientific advances, and life expectancy extending even longer? Or will new diseases and failing drugs cancel out these gains? If populations live longer, will these extra years be healthy and productive or merely an extended sentence of suffering? Will continuing population growth finally stifle the planet's life, depleting finite resources, polluting beyond repair, and making megacities and urban slums the home for more and more? Or will better family planning options – and mounting deaths from AIDS – reverse recent trends? Will we conquer malnutrition, obesity, drug abuse, poverty, depression and the common cold? Will we eradicate polio, leprosy, measles and other ancient foes? Will deaths from heart disease and cancer finally begin to decline? And when science surely delivers spectacular new therapeutic tools, who will be able to afford them? Will the gaps between the health of rich and poor grow ever wider?

If you are interested in reading more about mapping, you might like to look at the following:

- Monmonier, M. (1996) *How to Lie with Maps*. University of Chicago Press: Chicago. This illustrated essay on the use and abuse of maps teaches how to evaluate maps critically, and promotes a healthy scepticism about these easy-to-manipulate models of reality. It shows that despite their immense value, maps do, and in fact sometimes need, to lie.
- Dorling, D. and Fairbairn, D. (1997) *Mapping: Ways of Representing the World*. Longman: London.
- Dorling, D. (1996) *Area Cartograms: Their Use and Creation*. No. 59 Concepts and Techniques in Modern Geography (CATMOG), School of Environmental Sciences, University of East Anglia: Norwich.

Suggested activities

- Think critically, try to look at the world in a different way. How would you design a book like this or produce a newspaper story about a health incident? Suppose that you were able to produce a television documentary or film on health and society. How would you go about the work? All these forms of media are just the creation of people like you.
- If you are ever in London, go to Broadwick Street in Soho (formerly Broad Street) and have a look at the replica of the infamous pump. What is the area like today? How does it compare with other parts of London? Think about the interactions of health, place and society over a drink at the John Snow pub!
- Write a critical review of this book (aim for 800 words). By the time you are reading this some reviews may well have already been published in journals and you could look at those for ideas. What could we have done to have produced a better book? What are the most significant errors that we have made? What have we left out which we shouldn't have?

References

Cliff, A. and Haggett, P. (1988) *Atlas of Disease Distributions, Analytical Approaches to Epidemiological Data*. Blackwell: Oxford.

Chadwick, E. (1842) *Report from the Poor Law Commissioners on an Inquiry on the Sanitary Conditions of the Labouring Population of Great Britain*. HMSO: London (reprinted in 1965).

Dean, A.G. (1976) Population-based spot maps: an epidemiologic technique. *American Journal of Public Health*, 66(10): 988–9.

Dorling, D. (1995) *A New Social Atlas of Britain*. Wiley: Chichester.

Dorling, D. (1997) *Death in Britain: How Local Mortality Rates Have Changed: 1950s–1990s*. Joseph Rowntree Foundation: York.

Dorling, D. (1998) Mapping Disease Patterns. In *The Encyclopedia of Biostatistics*. Wiley: Chichester.

Engels, F. (1844; reprinted 1987) *The Condition of the Working Class in England*. Penguin: London.

Factory Inquiry Commission Report (1833) Parliamentary Papers.

Forster, F. (1966) Use of a demographic base map for the presentation of areal data in epidemiology. *British Journal of Preventative and Social Medicine*, 20: 165–71.

Howe, G.M. (1970) *National Atlas of Disease Mortality in the United Kingdom*, revised and enlarged edition. Thomas Nelson and Sons: London.

Krieger, N., Zapata, C., Murrain, M., Barnett, E., Parsons, P.E. and Birn, A. (1997) Spirit of 1848: a network linking polities, passion, and public health. *Radical Statistics*, 66: 22–32.

Levison, M.E. and Haddon, W. (1965) The area adjusted map: an epidemiological device. *Public Health Reports*, 80(1): 55–9.

Mitchell, R., Dorling, D. and Shaw, M. (2000) *Inequalities in Life and Death: What if Britain were More Equal?* The Policy Press: Bristol.

Rip, M.M., Paneth, N., Vinten-Johansen, P., Brody, H., Rachman, S. (1998) Cartpathology: John Snow and the London cholera epidemics 1848 and 1854 re-examined. *Proceedings of the Eighth International Symposium in Medical Geography*, Baltimore, Maryland, 13–17 July.

Robinson, A.H. (1982) *Early Thematic Mapping in the History of Cartography*. University of Chicago Press: Chicago.

Selvin, S., Merrill, D., Sacks, S., Wong, L., Bedell, L. and Schulman, J. (1984) *Transformations of Maps to Investigate Clusters of Disease*, Lawrence Berkeley Lab. Report, LBL-18550.

Selvin, S., Shaw, G., Schulman, J. and Merrill, D. (1987) Spatial distribution of disease: three case studies. *Journal of the National Cancer Institute*, 79(3): 417–23.

Selvin, S., Merrill, D., Schulman, J., Sacks, S., Bedell, L. and Wong, L. (1988) Transformations of maps to investigate clusters of diseases. *Social Science and Medicine*, 26(2): 215–21.

Shaw, M. and Dorling, D. (1998) Mortality among street sleeping youth in the UK. *The Lancet*, 352(9129): 743.

Snow, J. (1854) *On the Mode of Communication of Cholera*. Churchill Livingstone: London.

Stamp, L.D. (1962) A geographer's postscript. In D. Nichols (ed.) *Taxonomy and Geography*. The Systematics Association: London, 153–8.

Taylor, I. (1955) An epidemiology map. *Ministry of Health Monthly Bulletin*, 14, 200–1.

Tufte, E.R. (1997) *Visual Explanations: Images and Quantities, Evidence and Narrative*. Graphics Press: Cheshire, CT.

Wallace, J.M. (1926) Population map for health officers. *American Journal of Public Health*, 16(10): 1023.

Index

vaccination 25, 27, 96
values 36
  see also moral attitudes
variables 43–52, 69
  clinical characteristics 51–2
  confounding 112
  defined 43, 105
  key 45–8
    see also age; sex; wealth
  life course perspectives 48–9
  recording 69
  unemployment 49, 50
  see also data; dependent variables;
      independent variables; life expectancy;
      outcome
violence 146
  see also external causes

Wagar, W. 206
Wald, N. 44
Wales 115, 117
Wallace, D. and R. 83
Wallace, J.M. 193, 194
Ward, A. 13
waste disposal 22–3
  sanitation and sewage 24, 27, 28
water supply 23, 27–8
  and disease *see* cholera; diarrhoea
  pollution 23, 28
  pump on Broad Street 185, 187–8, 189,
      207
Watson, P. 110
wealth 3, 47–8
  accumulation of 164–5, 167

and inequalities 128, 129, 145, 150–1
  national, measures of 150
    see also GDP
weighting defined 113
welfare state 145
  see also NHS
Whitley, E. 34, 81, 83
WHO (World Health Organization)
  definition of health 25
  on future 206
  on maternal mortality 99
  on pollution 104
whooping cough 27
Wiencke, J.K. 44
Wilkinson, R.G. 89, 90, 150–1, 154
Williams, P. 59
Willis, P. 180
Wilm's tumour in New York State 198–9,
    205
Wohl, A.S. 37
Wolf, S. 120–1
women
  diet inadequate 23–4
  low status 100
  maternal mortality 96, 99–100
  medical practitioners 26, 36
  mortality in Scotland 195
  voting rights 158
  see also gender; sex
Woods, R. 23
working class 20, 21, 162, 180
World Health Organization *see* WHO

zipcodes 53–4